HANDBOOK OF
Zoonoses

IDENTIFICATION
AND PREVENTION

HANDBOOK OF
Zoonoses
IDENTIFICATION AND PREVENTION

JOANN L. COLVILLE, DVM

North Dakota State University, retired
Fargo, North Dakota

DAVID L. BERRYHILL, PhD

Director of Special Programs
College of Agriculture, Food Systems, and Natural Resources
Associate Professor, Department of Animal and Range Sciences
North Dakota State University
Fargo, North Dakota

With 60 illustrations

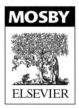

MOSBY
ELSEVIER

11830 Westline Industrial Drive
St. Louis, Missouri 63146

HANDBOOK OF ZOONOSES: ISBN: 978-0-323-04478-3
IDENTIFICATION AND PREVENTION
Copyright © 2007 by Mosby, Inc., an affiliate of Elsevier Inc.

Notice

Knowledge and best practice in this field are constantly changing. As new research and experience broaden our knowledge, changes in practice, treatment and drug therapy may become necessary or appropriate. Readers are advised to check the most current information provided (i) on procedures featured or (ii) by the manufacturer of each product to be administered, to verify the recommended dose or formula, the method and duration of administration, and contraindications. It is the responsibility of the practitioner, relying on their own experience and knowledge of the patient, to make diagnoses, to determine dosages and the best treatment for each individual patient, and to take all appropriate safety precautions. To the fullest extent of the law, neither the Publisher nor the Authors assume any liability for any injury and/or damage to persons or property arising out of or related to any use of the material contained in this book.

The Publisher

Library of Congress Control Number: 2007925084

Acquisitions Editor: Teri Merchant
Publishing Services Manager: Pat Joiner
Project Manager: Gena Magouirk
Cover Design Direction: Paula Ruckenbrod
Interior Design: Paula Ruckenbrod

Working together to grow
libraries in developing countries

www.elsevier.com | www.bookaid.org | www.sabre.org

ELSEVIER   BOOK AID International   Sabre Foundation

Printed in the United States of America.

Last digit is the print number: 9 8 7 6 5 4 3 2 1

To Tom, my "idea guy," who was always there with comments and suggestions, and to Audra, my "memory chick," who kept me on track when I would have gone elsewhere
JLC

To my parents
DLB

foreword

This book is written by a clinical veterinarian and clinical microbiologist and specifically designed for veterinarians, veterinary technicians, professional students, and healthcare professionals to help them understand and manage zoonotic diseases. The topic of zoonoses can be ripped from the current news headlines with such examples as West Nile virus, avian flu, *E. coli* gastroenteritis, toxoplasmosis, and anthrax, to name a few. Anthrax has received special attention in the news recently because of the possible use as a biological warfare agent. Veterinarians and technicians play a special role in the dissemination of current reliable veterinary medical information.

The general public has become dependent on the veterinary medical profession for the most current and accurate information on zoonoses. There are more than 150 diseases that are known to be zoonotic. This book provides a condensed source of clear, accurate, and easily accessible information about diseases that could potentially spread between patients, clients, and staff in a veterinary practice.

Each disease is systematically presented by giving accurate information on morbidity, mortality, etiology, hosts, transmission, virulence factors, clinical signs (animal and human), diagnosis, treatment, prevention, and control. Two summary boxes in Chapter One provide a quick reference to zoonotic diseases by etiology (viral, bacterial, fungal, parasitic) and zoonotic diseases by host (human, dogs, cats, cattle, horses, swine, sheep, goats, birds, rodents, snakes, and fish).

To be able to provide current zoonotic information to clients, staff, healthcare professionals, professional students, and the general public, this handbook is your reliable, quick resource to commonly sought-after information. This book provides current information on the hot topic of zoonoses in both veterinary medicine and human medicine.

Dennis M. McCurnin, DVM, MS, DACVS
Professor of Surgery
School of Veterinary Medicine
Louisiana State University
Baton Rouge, Louisiana

preface

We wrote this handbook to provide a source of basic information about zoonotic diseases—diseases that are transmitted from animals to humans. It is meant to be an easy-to-read and easy-to-understand handbook for quick reference and not an all-inclusive textbook about zoonoses. This handbook is intended for use by healthcare students and personnel on both the veterinary and human sides of medicine, but it is appropriate for those who are not in the healthcare industry as well.

Healthcare providers need this easy-to-use reference when presented with questions about diseases that may potentially travel between humans and other animals. There is common misinformation about some zoonotic diseases and a general lack of knowledge about other zoonotic diseases, especially diseases that have recently emerged. This book provides a clear, accurate, and easily accessible source of information about diseases that could potentially spread between veterinary patients, clients, and staff. The large body of knowledge about zoonoses has been carefully distilled down to the important nuggets of information that healthcare providers and the animal-owning public need to protect themselves, their patients, their clients, and their animals.

We have concentrated on how a zoonotic disease affects hosts, how it is spread, and what healthcare professionals need to know to provide correct information.

For readers who may not be familiar with some of the medical terms used, we have included a glossary. The diseases are listed in alphabetical order so they can be found easily. There are two boxes included that list the diseases by etiology and by host and a table that lists diseases by means of transmission. The diagrams that accompany some of the diseases illustrate how the diseases travel from infected animals to humans. For parasitic diseases, we have omitted parts of the parasitic life cycle in order to simplify the diagrams. Specific treatment regimens have not been included because there may be many treatments available for a single disease, and the drug(s) of choice for treatment of a disease may change.

A word of caution about quick references: The World Wide Web has become the "authoritative" source of information on just about every topic imaginable. Anyone can post information on a website, but the information isn't always accurate. We have gone through many reference books, textbooks, and websites to gather the information included in this handbook. To the best of our knowledge, all of the information included is accurate.

Joann L. Colville
David L. Berryhill

contents

Handbook of
Zoonoses
Identification and Prevention

PRINCIPLES OF ZOONOSES

one

INTRODUCTION

When people think about diseases they can get from animals, probably one of the first diseases that comes to mind is rabies. Indeed, rabies is a serious disease that has been around since before recorded history, but the chances of someone in North America developing rabies is pretty low. There are far more common diseases that we get from animals that do not get the attention or generate headlines as does rabies. Cat scratch fever affects over 20,000 people per year in the United States. Between 4% and 20% of children in America are infected with roundworms that have been transmitted from small animals. Compare that with the zero to four cases of rabies seen in the United States each year. Granted, unprotected people will die if they develop rabies, but cat scratch fever and roundworms can also cause death and have serious economic effects.

ZOONOTIC DISEASES

Zoonoses (singular: *zoonosis*; adjective: *zoonotic*) are diseases transmitted among humans and other vertebrates. The key word here is *among*. Zoonotic diseases can be transmitted from *nonhuman* animals (henceforth referred to as *animals*) to humans or from humans to animals. In this book the term *zoonotic disease* will refer to *diseases transmitted from animals to humans*.

Zoonotic diseases are not rare:

- All known microbial and parasitic categories include at least one zoonotic agent. From the smallest virus to the largest parasitic worm, there are many agents of disease, called *pathogens*, that can pass among people and animals (Box 1).
- A majority of infectious diseases are zoonotic. There are more than 150 diseases that are known to be zoonotic.
- Many human diseases probably started out as zoonotic diseases. Although we cannot be sure which diseases made the leap from animals to humans, there is evidence that measles, smallpox, and diphtheria came to us from animals. There is also compelling evidence that AIDS started in monkeys.
- About three quarters of emerging diseases are zoonotic, and when they appear, they can spread rapidly. The West Nile virus appeared in New York City in the United States in 1999 and moved through the country in the summer of 2002, causing human and equine disease and death.
- Most of the animals we come in contact with every day can be sources of zoonotic diseases (Box 2).

Reverse zoonoses are diseases that people can give to animals. Among the more common diseases are *Staphylococcus aureus* infection, *Streptococcus* infection, and tuberculosis.

There are diseases that people and animals share but that they do not get from each other. For example, blastomycosis and coccidioidomycosis are nonzoonotic *mycotic* (fungal) diseases that people and animals develop from exposure to contaminated soil but not from exposure to each other.

And then there are the diseases that people think they can get from animals, but it just does not happen. These *pseudozoonotic* diseases include feline leukemia; feline immunodeficiency disease, also known as *feline AIDS;* pinworms; colds; and sore throats.

Box 1. Zoonotic diseases grouped by etiology

VIRAL DISEASES
Eastern equine encephalitis
Hantavirus pulmonary syndrome
Influenza
La Crosse encephalitis
Lymphocytic choriomeningitis
Rabies
St. Louis encephalitis
West Nile virus infections
Western equine encephalitis

BACTERIAL DISEASES
Anthrax
Botulism
Brucellosis
Campylobacteriosis
Cat scratch disease
Colibacillosis
Ehrlichiosis
Leptospirosis
Listeriosis
Lyme disease
Mycobacterial infections
Pasteurellosis
Plague
Psittacosis
Q fever
Rat-bite fever
Rocky Mountain spotted fever
Salmonellosis

Staphylococcosis
Tularemia
Vibriosis
Yersiniosis

FUNGAL DISEASE
Dermatomycosis

PARASITIC DISEASES
Arthropod infestation
    Scabies
Protozoan infections
    Babesiosis
    Cryptosporidiosis
    Giardiasis
    Toxoplasmosis
Round worm infections
    Cutaneous larva migrans
    Heartworm infection
    Hookworm infection
    Roundworm infection
    Trichinellosis
    Visceral larva migrans
Tapeworm infections
    Diphyllobothriasis
    Dipylidiasis
    Echinococcosis

PRION DISEASE
Bovine spongiform encephalopathy

BOX 2. Zoonotic diseases grouped by host

DOGS
Brucellosis
Campylobacteriosis
Cryptosporidiosis
Giardiasis
Hookworm infection
Leptospirosis
Lyme disease
Q fever
Rabies
Ringworm infection
Roundworm *(Toxocara)* infection
Rocky Mountain spotted fever
Salmonellosis
Tapeworm *(Dipylidium)* infection

CATS
Campylobacteriosis
Cat scratch disease *(Bartonella henselae* infection)
Cryptosporidiosis
Hookworm infection
Leptospirosis
Plague *(Yersinia pestis* infection)
Q fever
Rabies
Ringworm infection
Roundworm *(Toxocara)* infection
Salmonellosis
Tapeworm *(Dipylidium)* infection
Toxoplasmosis

CATTLE
Anthrax
Bovine spongiform encephalopathy
Brucellosis
Campylobacteriosis
Cryptosporidiosis

Colibacillosis
Q fever
Rabies
Ringworm infection
Salmonellosis

HORSES
Campylobacteriosis
Cryptosporidiosis
Leptospirosis
Rabies
Ringworm infection
Salmonellosis

SWINE
Q fever
Ringworm infection
Yersiniosis

SHEEP AND GOATS
Anthrax
Q fever

BIRDS
Campylobacteriosis
Psittacosis *(Chlamydophila psittaci* infection)
Salmonellosis

RODENTS
Hantavirus pulmonary syndrome
Lymphocytic choriomeningitis
Rat-bite fever
Salmonellosis

SNAKES
Salmonellosis

Continued

Box 2. Zoonotic diseases grouped by host—cont'd

FISH
Salmonellosis

WILDLIFE
Anthrax
Brucellosis
Giardiasis
Hantavirus pulmonary syndrome

Lymphocytic choriomeningitis
Plague (*Yersinia pestis* infection)
Rabies
Roundworm infection, racoon
  (*Baylisascaris* infection)
Tuberculosis (*Mycobacterium* infection)
Tularemia (*Francisella tularensis*
  infection)

HOSTS

People are often accidental and dead-end hosts for zoonotic diseases. The definitive host of a pathogen is also the natural host of the pathogen. In the case of zoonotic diseases, the definitive hosts are animals. Sometimes definitive hosts become ill from the pathogens, and sometimes they do not. If the animal does not become ill but is still capable of transmitting the disease to people, it is said to be a *carrier*, or *reservoir host*. Carriers can also be inanimate objects, such as water or food.

MODES OF TRANSMISSION

There are a number of methods used to transmit diseases from animals to people. The two major categories of transmission are direct transmission and indirect transmission (Table 1).

DIRECT TRANSMISSION

Contact between the infected animal and the susceptible person can result in *direct transmission* of a zoonotic disease. This can take place by touching the animal or from droplet infection through the animal's coughing or sneezing.

TABLE 1.   Zoonotic diseases identified by typical means of transmission

DISEASE	BITE/ SCRATCH	CONTACT	INGESTION	INHALATION	INSECT VECTOR
Anthrax		X	X	X	
Babesiosis					X
Botulism			X		
Bovine spongiform encephalopathy			X		
Brucellosis		X	X		
Campylobacteriosis		X	X		
Cat scratch disease	X				
Colibacillosis			X		
Cryptosporidiosis			X		
Dermatomycosis		X			
Eastern equine encephalitis					X
Ehrlichiosis					X
Giardiasis			X		
Hantavirus pulmonary syndrome				X	
Hookworm infection		X	X		
Influenza		X		X	

TABLE 1.   Zoonotic diseases identified by typical means
of transmission—cont'd

DISEASE	BITE/ SCRATCH	CONTACT	INGESTION	INHALATION	INSECT VECTOR
La Crosse encephalitis					X
Leptospirosis		X	X		
Listeriosis			X		
Lyme disease					X
Lymphocytic choriomeningitis		X	X	X	
Mycobacterium infection (Tuberculosis)		X	X	X	
Pasteurellosis	X				
Plague		X		X	X
Psittacosis				X	
Q fever				X	
Rabies	X				
Rat-bite fever	X		X		
Rocky Mountain spotted fever					X
Roundworm infection			X		
St. Louis encephalitis					X
Salmonellosis			X		
Scabies		X			
Staphylococcosis			X		
Tapeworm infection			X		
Toxoplasmosis			X		
Trichinosis			X		
Tularemia		X	X	X	X
Vibriosis		X	X		
West Nile virus infection					X
Western equine encephalitis					X
Yersiniosis			X		

A person must be within 1 meter in front of an animal for direct droplet transmission to occur. The pathogen may stay on the person's skin, enter the body through breaks in the skin or mucosal surfaces, be ingested, or be inhaled. Plague is an example of a disease contracted via direct transmission.

INDIRECT TRANSMISSION

Indirect transmission includes any method of transmission in which the infected animal and susceptible person do not actually come in direct contact. Some of these methods include:

- Transmission that involves contact between the person and some inanimate object known as a *fomite*. Animals contaminate objects with pathogens, and people become infected when they come in contact with the contaminated objects. One example is *dermatophytes,* fungi that cause skin infections that can be transmitted to people via contact with contaminated bedding, grooming tools, etc. Another example is dust particles contaminated with a pathogen that can enter a person through the respiratory tract, such as with *Hantavirus* infection. As with direct transmission, any pathogen acquired through indirect transmission may stay on the person's skin, enter the body through breaks in the skin or mucosal surfaces, be ingested, or be inhaled. Examples of *fomites* include grooming utensils, blankets, clothing, toys, and dust particles.
- Indirect transmission can also involve *vectors*. There are two types of vectors—*biological vectors* and *mechanical vectors:*
  - *Biological vectors* are animals in which the pathogen must go through part of its life cycle before being passed on to a person. Examples of biological vectors are fleas, ticks, flies, and mosquitoes. They can be reservoir hosts for a pathogen, as in babesiosis.
  - *Mechanical vectors* are animals that carry pathogens to people but are not themselves affected by the pathogens. Examples of mechanical vectors are mosquitoes, ticks, flies, and pets. Yes, insects and arthropods can be either biological or mechanical vectors. They can also be carrier hosts for a pathogen. For example, flies can spread salmonellosis with their feet.
- *Vehicles of transmission* are neither fomites nor vectors. They are substances that are normally brought into the body upon which a pathogen has hitched a ride. Vehicles include water, air, and food. When water is a vehicle of transmission, it is usually contaminated with feces from an infected animal, as in giardiasis. Air can be a vehicle if the person is standing more than 1 meter away from an infected animal when it sneezes or coughs and the pathogen becomes airborne on dust particles or in droplets. Food transmission usually results in food poisoning.

PREVENTING ZOONOTIC DISEASES

Except for smallpox vaccination, few tools for protecting people and animals from zoonotic diseases were available before the early 1900s. Methods such as thoroughly cooking meat, boiling milk, and quarantining sick animals were used to control diseases. In the 1920s commercial pasteurization became an effective way to prevent zoonotic diseases that are spread through raw milk or products made from raw milk. Insecticides came into use in the 1940s and helped protect against vector-borne diseases. Vaccines are available to protect animals and people against some zoonotic diseases but not all of them. In the 1950s, the United States started mandatory vaccination of dogs for rabies, and that has been a primary contributing factor in the decline in the number of rabies cases seen in people.

ABOUT THE DISEASES

In the next section of this book, you will be introduced to many of the known zoonotic diseases. The diseases are listed in alphabetical order by their most commonly used names. Sometimes that means using a common name (cat scratch disease) instead of the etiologic name (bartonellosis). Other times we use the etiologic name (listeriosis) rather than the common name (silage disease) because it is more frequently used. Each disease section contains a description of the disease's etiology; its hosts; its mode(s) of transmission; methods for diagnosis, treatment, and prevention; and other useful information.

MORBIDITY AND MORTALITY

At the beginning of each disease section, a scale of 1 to 4 plus marks (+ to ++++) indicates the morbidity and mortality for the disease. The *morbidity* is the likelihood that a person will contract the disease. The *mortality* is the likelihood that a person who has developed the disease will die as a result.

ZOONOTIC DISEASES two

ANTHRAX

Anthrax occurs worldwide. It is usually seen in areas where animals have died from anthrax and contaminated the soil with spores. Outbreaks of anthrax are most often associated with warm weather seasons, heavy rains, and/or droughts.

MORBIDITY: +
MORTALITY: + TO ++++
ETIOLOGY: BACTERIAL

Anthrax is caused by *Bacillus anthracis*, a gram-positive, encapsulated, spore-forming aerobic rod. The organism exists in two forms: the *vegetative form*, which causes disease, and the *sporulated form*, which is dormant. Oxygen is needed for sporulation (development from the vegetative state into spores). Spores are usually found in the soil and can lay dormant for decades.

HOSTS

Most mammals, including humans, are susceptible to anthrax infection to some degree. Ruminants such as cattle, sheep, and goats are most commonly infected because they are grazing animals and may graze on grass growing in infected soil. Other herbivores like horses and pigs may also be infected. Anthrax has been reported in dogs and cats but is rare in these animals.

TRANSMISSION

Humans are infected by ingestion or inhalation of anthrax spores or by handling contaminated carcasses, wool, hide, or hair (Figure 1). When a person is infected through handling a contaminated object, the spores enter through preexisting skin cuts or abrasions. Direct person-to-person spread of anthrax is extremely rare. Communicability is not a concern in managing or visiting with patients with inhalational anthrax.

In animals, the most common form of transmission is ingestion of anthrax spores. The spores in the soil are ingested when environmental conditions are right. Periods of heavy rain can wash the spores into low-lying areas, where they are exposed to oxygen as they are brought to the surface, and animals

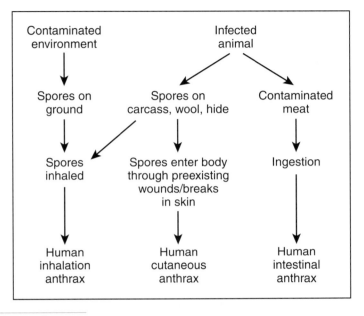

FIGURE 1. Anthrax

grazing in these areas ingest the spores. Drought conditions, in which pastures have little plant growth, can also be a contributing factor. Animals graze closer to the ground than they normally would and may ingest spores. Biting flies can, but rarely do, transmit *B. anthracis* from one animal to another. Outbreaks in pigs have been associated with feed containing meat and/or bone meal from infected carcasses. Wild animals or other scavengers become infected by feeding on infected dead animals.

VIRULENCE FACTORS

All virulent strains of *B. anthracis* form a nontoxic capsule that functions to protect the organism against the bactericidal components of plasma and phagocytes and against destruction by gastric juices.

An exotoxin plays a major role in the pathogenesis of anthrax. One component of the anthrax toxin has a lethal mode of action that is not understood at this time. Death is apparently due to oxygen depletion, secondary shock, and respiratory and cardiac failure. Death from anthrax in humans or animals frequently occurs suddenly and unexpectedly.

ANTHRAX IN ANIMALS

CATTLE, SHEEP, AND GOATS

Anthrax in ruminants may cause a peracute (very sudden) disease, in which the animals are found dead, having shown no clinical signs before death. The carcasses are bloated, with little or no rigor mortis and bloody discharges that do not clot coming from body openings. Acute cases of anthrax are associated with sudden illness, characterized by high fever, localized edema (in more longstanding cases), decreased or absent rumination, decreased milk production with blood-tinged or yellow-colored milk, excitement followed by depression, difficult breathing, convulsions, bleeding that does not clot coming from body openings, and death. Anthrax can cause abortion. The incubation period is 1 to 3 days following exposure, with death usually occuring in 2 to 3 days.

HORSES

Horses can become infected with anthrax either through ingestion or through the bite of an insect. If a horse is infected through ingestion, the resulting disease is sudden and is characterized by loss of appetite, colic, bloody diarrhea, fever, and death in 2 to 4 days. Insect bites produce localized swelling around the bite wound and edema in the lower parts of the body.

PIGS

Pigs are relatively resistant to anthrax infection, but when infected will most often develop edema in their throats and subsequently suffocate. Some animals will recover in a couple of days.

CATS AND DOGS

Anthrax is rarely reported in cats and dogs because they seem to be relatively resistant to infection. When anthrax is seen, it is most often the gastrointestinal form of the disease resulting from eating infected meat or hides. Cats can become infected by grooming themselves if their fur is contaminated with spores. Ulcers may form in the mouth and throat, and edema may develop around the head and neck regions. The incubation period may be as long as 2 weeks. Some animals die suddenly without exhibiting any clinical signs.

ANTHRAX IN HUMANS

Three forms of anthrax are seen in humans.

CUTANEOUS FORM

The cutaneous form is the most common, accounting for nearly 95% of all human anthrax cases. The incubation period is 1 to 12 days, and the disease is characterized by what initially looks like an insect bite. Localized, painless ulceration with a central black scab (Figure 2); fever; and headache develop rapidly. These symptoms may be followed within a few days by septicemia and meningitis. There is a 20% fatality rate if the disease is left untreated.

PULMONARY OR INHALATION FORM

The pulmonary, or inhalation, form (also known as *woolsorter's disease*) is caused by inhalation of spores from contaminated carcasses, wool, hide, or hair. The spores may also be found on brush bristles, after grooming an animal with contaminated fur. The incubation period is 1 to 5 days, up to a month and a half. The disease may initially present as a cold or the flu. It is characterized by fever, sore throat, nonproductive cough, difficulty breathing, muscle aches, respiratory failure, and usually death within 24 hours. Mortality can reach 95% if treatment is not started within 2 days.

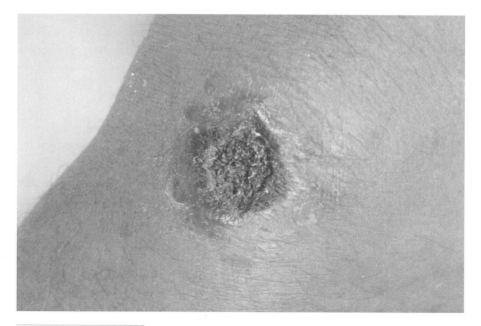

FIGURE 2. Cutaneous anthrax with central dark scab. (Courtesy Public Health Image Library, PHIL 2033, Centers for Disease Control and Prevention, Atlanta, 1962, James H. Steele.)

INTESTINAL OR GASTROINTESTINAL FORM

The intestinal or gastrointestinal form results from ingestion of contaminated meat. This form is rare in the United States. The incubation period is 12 hours to 5 days. Fever, anorexia, nausea, vomiting, and diarrhea are followed by intestinal pain and vomiting blood. Mortality averages around 50% if untreated.

DIAGNOSIS

A tentative diagnosis in some animals, primarily ruminants, can be made from the physical signs found on a carcass; the sudden death, accompanied by bloody discharges that do not clot coming from body openings; and incomplete or no rigor mortis. Sputum, blood, or tissue can be Gram stained to look for gram-positive rods. Culture on blood agar yields nonmotile, nonhemolytic, bacterial colonies. Antibody titers will be elevated. Chest radiographs are taken in people suspected of having inhalation anthrax.

TREATMENT

The U.S. Food and Drug Administration (FDA) has approved penicillin, ciprofloxacin, and doxycycline for treatment of anthrax in humans. Penicillin and tetracycline are used in animals. There are different strains of *B. anthracis*; some strains will be resistant to one antibiotic but not another. Resistant strains of *B. anthracis* could be developed and manufactured as biological weapons.

PREVENTION

An anthrax vaccine is available for livestock, but none has been approved for use in cats and dogs. Animal vaccines cannot be used in humans.

An anthrax vaccine has been licensed for use in high-risk humans. The vaccine is reported to be 93% effective if boostered annually. Pregnant women should be vaccinated only if absolutely necessary.

CONTROL

Anthrax in both animals and humans is a reportable disease in the United States. Infections must be reported to local, state, and federal animal health officials. If you are submitting samples to a diagnostic laboratory, ask the laboratory what samples are required and be sure to inform the laboratory of a possible anthrax infection.

If an animal is found dead or dies following treatment and anthrax is suspected, leave the carcass alone. Do not touch it, and do not open it for a necropsy. Doing so will release vegetative *B. anthracis* that will convert to spores when exposed to the air and contaminate the immediate environment. In humans this may result in an inhalation or cutaneous anthrax infection. Notify a veterinarian who will dispose of the carcass. Carcasses will be burned where they are found and/or buried at least 4 feet deep (some states require burying 10 feet deep) and covered with lime. The soil directly under the carcass will be burned and buried also.

If an animal is diagnosed with anthrax, the herd from which it came will be quarantined. Exposed animals that look healthy will be vaccinated. Animals that appear sick will be isolated and treated. The pasture where the animals are feeding will be abandoned if possible. Animals that have recently left the herd will be located, and the premises where they currently reside quarantined. When the disease is under control, the premises need to be cleaned.

Preventing cats and dogs from scavenging on carcasses, especially if the cause of death is unknown, will prevent them from getting infected.

ANTHRAX AND BIOLOGICAL WARFARE

The possibility of creating aerosols of anthrax spores has made *B. anthracis* a potential biological weapon. Spores of *B. anthracis* can be produced and stored in a dry form, and they remain viable for decades in storage or after release.

A cloud of anthrax spores could be released at a strategic location and inhaled by the individuals under attack. An infection of local animal populations could follow the attack. Infected animals could then transmit the disease to humans through cutaneous, intestinal, or inhalation routes.

HISTORICAL NOTE

In 1877, *B. anthracis* was the first bacterium shown to be the cause of a disease. Robert Koch grew the organism and injected it into animals, and the animals developed anthrax.

BABESIOSIS

Babesiosis is a parasitic infection of red blood cells that is spread by a tick bite. The disease is also known as piroplasmosis (*pirum* means *pear* in Greek) because the parasite appears pear-shaped in red blood cells. Human babesiosis is also known as *Nantucket fever* because the disease was first diagnosed after an outbreak on Nantucket Island, Massachusetts.

MORBIDITY: +

MORTALITY: +

ETIOLOGY: PARASITIC

Babesia microti causes most human infections in North America. *B. gibsoni* and *B. canis* cause babesiosis in dogs, and in horses *B. equi* and *B. caballi* are the causative species. *B. gibsoni*, *B. canis*, and *B. equi* have been identified in rare human infections. *B. equi* has been reclassified as *Theileria equi*, but the original name is still commonly used.

Babesia organisms invade red blood cells, causing their destruction when the *Babesia* organisms multiply within those cells.

HOSTS

The white-footed mouse is the primary host for *B. microti*, the species that most often infects people. This species has also been found in field mice, voles, rats, chipmunks, and cottontail rabbits. Horses are the host for *B. equi* and *B. caballi*. Dogs are the host for *B. gibsoni* and *B. canis*. In all cases a tick is the *vector*, meaning it is infected but not affected by the organism.

TRANSMISSION

Hard-bodied, or *ixodid*, ticks are vectors for babesiosis. The black-legged deer tick is the primary vector for *B. microti*, and the brown dog tick is the vector for *B. gibsoni* and *B. canis*. Many hard ticks can act as vectors for equine babesiosis. Ticks ingest *Babesia* while feeding off of an infected host, and the parasite enters the tick's digestive system, where it multiplies within the tick's intestinal wall. The parasites then travel to the tick's salivary glands, where they are passed to another host when the tick takes its next meal. Transmission can occur via the larva, nymph, or adult tick.

The deer tick life cycle takes an average of 2 years to complete. Female ticks lay their eggs on the ground in early spring. By summer, eggs hatch into larvae. Larvae prefer to feed on mice, other small mammals, and birds in the summer and early fall. They will then molt into nymphs and become inactive until spring. Cold weather (near or below freezing) inhibits tick activity. During the following spring and summer, nymphs will feed on white-footed mice or other rodents, birds, and other small mammals, and in the fall they will molt into adults. Most people are infected by nymphs. The adult ticks prefer to feed and mate on large animals, such as whitetail deer, in the fall and early spring. Female ticks then drop off of these animals and lay eggs on the ground, and a new life cycle begins (Figure 3).

After being deposited in a new host, the parasites invade red blood cells, multiply, and eventually rupture the membranes of infected red blood cells and invade other red blood cells (Figure 4).

With *B. microti*, the tick larvae and nymphs feed primarily on the white-footed deer mouse. The adult ticks feed on whitetail deer, which do not

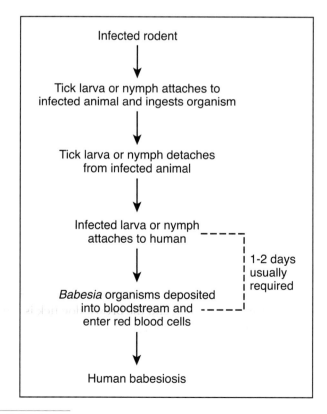

FIGURE 3.   Babesiosis.

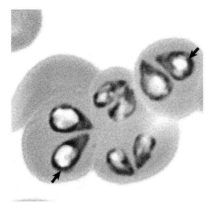

FIGURE 4.   *Babesia* organisms in red blood cells. (From Harvey JW: Atlas of veterinary hematology: blood and bone marrow of domestic animals, St Louis, 2001, Saunders.)

become infected with *B. microti*. The adult ticks mate while they are feeding on the deer, so even though the deer do not become infected, they allow the life cycle of the tick to continue. The parasite passes from larva to nymph to adult tick as the tick matures. Human infections are accidental occurrences. Person-to-person infections, via blood transfusions and transplacental infection, have been reported.

BABESIOSIS IN ANIMALS

DOGS

Babesiosis in dogs is a cyclical disease, in that recovery from the initial infection shows variable and unpredictable periods of illness, alternating with apparently healthy periods.

The clinical signs vary, depending on the stage of the disease and the age and immune status of the dog. Young animals are more severely affected than older animals. A tick must be attached to a susceptible host for 2 to 3 days before *Babesia* organisms are passed to the host. There can be three phases to canine babesiosis: acute, subclinical, and chronic.

The acute phase is the initial infection and usually lasts a short time. It is characterized by hemolytic anemia, enlarged lymph nodes, enlarged spleen, vomiting, lethargy, and fever. Most dogs recover after treatment.

The subclinical phase can last months or years. It is characterized by a balance between the *Babesia* organisms and the immune system of the host, so there is little clinical evidence of disease. The balance can be upset by stress, concurrent infections (especially ehrlichiosis), immunosuppression, removal of the spleen, surgery, or extreme exercise. During this phase, the dog may show only an intermittent fever and anorexia. When the balance is upset, the

Babesia organisms will begin to increase in number, and the dog will move into the next phase. Greyhounds are frequently subclinical carriers of babesiosis, and they can spread the disease through blood transfusions or to their puppies transplacentally.

The chronic phase begins if the dog is unable to clear the red blood cells containing the *Babesia* organisms from circulation. This phase is characterized by a cycle of lethargy, anorexia, and a gradual loss of body condition, seen most obviously along the spine and around the eyes. Other symptoms include coughing or labored breathing, vomiting, constipation or diarrhea, sores in the mouth, edema, abdominal swelling, a rash or bleeding under the skin, blood clotting problems, swollen joints, seizures, weakness, enlarged lymph nodes, enlarged spleen, and depression.

In rare cases, the central nervous system can be involved, resulting in weakness, incoordination, and seizures.

HORSES

B. caballi causes a less severe disease, because only about 1% of the red blood cells are infected. Infections may not be apparent but can persist 1 to 4 years before they are completely eliminated from the horse. *B. caballi* can be associated with anorexia, poor performance, and weight loss.

B. equi infects up to 20% of red blood cells, leading to more severe clinical signs including fever, anemia, jaundice, increased respiratory and heart rates, and an enlarged spleen. The parasites destroy red blood cells, resulting in hemolytic anemia. The hemoglobin released from the red blood cells may cause jaundice and dark urine. Colic, constipation followed by diarrhea, and swelling of the legs can occur. Foals can be infected transplacentally and can be aborted or born anemic and weak.

Subclinically infected animals can be carriers of the organism. Subclinical babesiosis may negatively affect the animal's performance. Strenuous exercise, such as racing, can cause subclinical infections to become acute. Geographic movement of apparently healthy horses may help spread *Babesia*.

BABESIOSIS IN HUMANS

Most people who are infected with *Babesia* never develop clinical disease. An infected tick must be attached to a person for at least 1 to 2 days before *Babesia* organisms are transmitted. Babesiosis will develop most often in people who are immunocompromised, have had their spleens removed, or are elderly. The spleen is one of the organs that is responsible for removing infected red blood cells from circulation, so if it is missing, the infected red blood cells stay in circulation, where the organism can infect more cells. Clinical signs of babesiosis will appear 1 to 4 weeks following a tick bite. They begin with flulike symptoms including fever, chills, and headache and progress to fatigue, anorexia, and muscle pain. Hemolytic anemia may develop, along with an enlarged liver and/or spleen. The hemolytic anemia may result in dark urine. The number of platelets circulating in blood may also be decreased, potentially causing bleeding disorders. Babesiosis in humans is rarely fatal, but death is seen more often in people who have had their spleens removed.

DIAGNOSIS

Diagnosis can be made by microscopic examination of stained blood smears to identify the organisms in red blood cells. Serological tests are available. Polymerase chain reaction (PCR) is a test that may also be used to detect *Babesia* DNA in the blood. Isolation of the organism by injection of patient blood into hamsters or gerbils may also assist in diagnosis. Animals inoculated with infective blood typically develop parasites in their red blood cells within 1 to 4 weeks.

TREATMENT

In humans, a combination of antimalarial drugs and antibiotics is used to treat babesiosis, along with symptomatic care. Dogs are treated with antibiotics. In all cases, the sooner treatment is begun, the more effective it will be.

PREVENTION

Tick and rodent control is the best approach to prevention. Avoiding endemic regions during the peak transmission months is especially important for people who have had their spleens removed or for immunocompromised persons, in whom babesiosis can be a devastating illness.

Tick-control products, such as tick collars, should be used on dogs that could possibly be exposed to ticks. This will help protect them from possible *Babesia* infection and will help decrease the number of ticks the dogs could possibly bring into a house, where people could be exposed to the ticks.

Decrease exposure to ticks by following these guidelines:
- Avoid areas where vector ticks thrive as much as possible. May, June, and July are the months when ticks are still immature and are harder to see because

of their light color. These are also the months when people are most active outdoors.

- Ticks have to live where their hosts live, so areas where white-footed mice and whitetail deer live are where ticks are found. These places can include lawns, gardens, wooded areas, overgrown brush, tall grass, woodpiles, and leaf litter.
- Wear light-colored clothing when entering an area that may be a habitat for ticks. This will make the adult ticks easier to see and remove before they become attached.
- Wear long-sleeved shirts and long pants tucked into socks so the ticks cannot crawl under clothing. Wear high, rubber boots and a hat for the same reason.
- Walk in the center of a trail to avoid vegetation, where ticks are lurking. Ticks cannot fly, jump, skip, or hop, so they must come in direct contact with a host before they can attach themselves. Immature ticks are found hiding in the shade, in moist areas. Adult ticks cling to grass, bushes, and shrubs and wait for a host to come by.
- Exposed skin and clothing can be protected with insect repellents containing N, N-diethyl-m-toluamide (DEET). Clothes, but not exposed skin, can be protected with insect repellents containing permethrin, which kills ticks on contact.
- Check often for ticks while outside. Black-legged ticks are tiny and easy to miss.
- Do not sit on the ground or on stone walls, where ticks abound.
- Make daily checks of the entire body for ticks. Look especially in areas where ticks like to attach, such as behind the ears, at the back of the neck, in the armpits, behind the knees, and in the groin area. Bathing will remove crawling ticks but will not detach ticks already attached. Daily tick checks and prompt removal of an attached tick are vital to reducing the risk of transmission.
- Wash outdoor clothing in hot water and dry at high temperatures after use.
- Remove ticks as soon as they are found. Remember it takes up to 2 days after a tick becomes attached before it starts transmitting *Babesia*.

To remove a tick, use fine tweezers, grasp the tick as close to the skin as possible, and pull straight back with a slow, steady force. Avoid crushing the tick's body. Kill the tick by dropping it in alcohol. Save the tick in alcohol as a possible diagnostic aid.

NOTE

Co-infection with *Borrelia burgdorferi* (Lyme disease) and *B. microti* may be relatively common in endemic areas of the United States. Co-infection with *Ehrlichia* species may also be seen.

BOTULISM

Among its more common names, botulism is also known as *limberneck* in birds and *shaker foal syndrome* in horses. Botulism is caused by the toxins (byproducts of bacterial growth) of *Clostridium botulinum*. The disease is characterized by progressive muscle paralysis, in which the muscles go flaccid or floppy. The paralysis can eventually affect cardiac and respiratory muscles, resulting in death. While the disease is relatively rare, the outcome can be devastating. The *C. botulinum* toxins are some of the most deadly poisons known. They could be used in a bioterrorist attack by aerosol dispersal or food and/or water contamination. One gram of crystallized *C. botulinum* toxin is enough to kill a million people.

MORBIDITY: +
MORTALITY: + TO ++++
ETIOLOGY: BACTERIAL NEUROTOXIN

Botulism is caused by toxins that attach themselves to the ends of nerves and interfere with the ability of the nerve to send impulses to muscles. The muscles become flaccid (muscle tone is absent), resulting in paralysis. The toxins are produced by the bacterium *C. botulinum*, an anaerobic, gram-positive, spore-forming, rod-shaped organism. It grows in an environment that is low in oxygen. If this condition is not available it produces spores, a dormant form of the organism that can survive in soil for a long time. When conditions are right, the spores will germinate and start growing, producing toxins. There are seven distinct toxins produced by *C. botulinum* that are designated by the first seven letters of the alphabet.

HOSTS

Many species of mammals, fish, and birds may be hosts.
- Types A, B, E, and F cause diseases in humans. Type A is found mostly west of the Mississippi River, type B is found in eastern states, and type E is found in Alaska and in the Great Lakes area.
- Type A is used to manufacture Botox for cosmetic and therapeutic purposes.
- Type B can cause disease in horses and cattle.
- Type C is the most common toxin to cause disease in animals. It is found most often in the western United States.

- Type D can cause disease in cattle and dogs. It is seen most often in South Africa, South America, and Australia.
- Types A and E are found in birds and mink.
- Type G rarely causes disease, but it has been associated with disease in humans.

TRANSMISSION

C. botulinum and *C. botulinum* spores are found in soil worldwide, in the intestinal tracts of mammals and fish, and in the gills and internal organs of shellfish. Transmission occurs when animals (including humans) ingest the toxins preformed by the bacteria or ingest the bacteria, which then start to produce toxins. Preformed toxins are found in decaying carcasses; decaying vegetable matter; and improperly home-canned foods (especially vegetables with low acid content, such as asparagus, green beans, beets, and corn) and fruits. They can also be found in improperly cooked beef, pork, poultry, and milk products. Transmission can also occur through a wound infection. Botulism is not spread directly between animals by casual contact, but an infected dead animal can be toxic if ingested by another animal. Maggots feeding on an infected carcass can also be a source of infection, if eaten by another animal.

BOTULISM IN ANIMALS

Botulism is seen most commonly in wild birds, domestic poultry, cattle, sheep, horses, and some species of fish. Pigs and dogs are relatively resistant to botulism. There have been no reported cases of botulism in cats.

Botulism in animals is generally associated with ingestion of preformed toxins that cause a progressive paralysis, resulting in a lack of muscle tone. The symptoms appear anywhere from 2 hours to 2 weeks after infection, but most often within 24 hours. Clinical signs include difficulty chewing and swallowing, visual impairment, and generalized weakness. The paralysis eventually may affect the muscles of the heart and lungs, resulting in death. A form of botulism called *toxicoinfectious botulism* results from eating the *C. botulinum* organism that then produces toxins in the gastrointestinal tract.

CATTLE

Botulism in cattle is usually associated with eating preformed toxins in contaminated feed. If small animals (mice, snakes, etc.) or animal carcasses are baled into hay or packed into silage, they could be a source of *C. botulinum* toxins at a later time, when the cattle are fed the hay or silage. Botulism is sometimes seen when cattle that are lacking phosphorus or protein in their diets eat carcass bones, with attached bits of meat, or soil to supply the lacking nutrients. Both the bones and the soil could be contaminated with *C. botulinum* toxins. Clinical signs of botulism include drooling and tongue paralysis, resulting in the tongue hanging out of the mouth; incoordination; difficulty eating; drooping eyelids; and lying down in a sternal position (lying on the chest). Weakness starts in the back legs and moves toward the head. If the animal goes into lateral recumbency (lying on its side), it is near death.

SHEEP
Clinical signs of botulism include drooling, clear nasal discharge, incoordination, and stiffness.

HORSES
Botulism in horses is similar to botulism in cattle. Horses can develop three types of botulism:
- Forage poisoning from ingestion of preformed *C. botulinum* toxins
- Toxicoinfectious disease from ingestion of the *C. botulinum* organism
- Wound botulism from wound infection

Clinical signs of botulism include restlessness, incoordination, tongue paralysis, and sternal recumbence. The muscle paralysis usually starts in the back legs and progresses to the front legs, neck, and head. *Shaker foal syndrome* is a condition seen in foals less than 4 weeks old. The foal may be found dead without having exhibited any clinical signs of illness. If clinical signs are present, they show up as a progressive, symmetrical paralysis, accompanied by a stiff gait, muscle tremors, and the inability to stand for more than 4 to 5 minutes. The foal may have difficulty eating, constipation, dilated pupils, and frequent urination. Death usually occurs 24 to 72 hours after the appearance of clinical signs.

BIRDS
In both domestic poultry and wild fowl, botulism is seen as paralysis of the legs, wings, neck, and eyelids. Water birds with paralyzed necks (hence the name *limberneck*) can drown. Some domestic broiler chickens have developed toxicoinfectious disease, from ingestion of the *C. botulinum* organisms. These birds will have diarrhea.

PIGS
Pigs are relatively resistant to botulism. If they get sick, the symptoms include lack of appetite, lack of desire to drink water, vomiting, dilated pupils, and paralysis.

DOGS

Although dogs are relatively resistant to botulism, they can come in contact with the C. botulinum toxin if they are allowed to eat infected, dead animals. The amount of toxin ingested will determine the severity of the disease. The most obvious clinical sign is extreme weakness, seen from a few hours to several days after ingestion of the toxin. The dogs cannot stand, but they are alert and can wag their tails.

BOTULISM IN HUMANS

There are three forms of botulism in humans: foodborne botulism, wound botulism, and infant botulism. In *foodborne botulism*, toxins are preformed in contaminated food and ingested when the food is eaten. In both *wound botulism* and *infant botulism*, the C. botulinum organism is present in a wound or in the large intestine of an infant and produces the toxin in vivo. All three forms can be fatal. If botulism is suspected, it should be treated as a medical emergency.

FOODBORNE BOTULISM

About one fourth of the cases of botulism reported annually in the United States are foodborne. The most common source of foodborne botulism is home-canned food that is not adequately heated during the canning or food preparation process. Adequate heat is necessary to kill the spores of C. botulinum so they cannot germinate and produce toxins in the canned foods. The clinical signs of foodborne botulism usually appear within 12 to 36 hours following ingestion of the toxin in contaminated food. The incubation period may be as long as a week or more. There is no fever associated with foodborne botulism, but nausea, vomiting, abdominal cramping, and diarrhea may appear before the neurological signs. When the neurological signs appear, they start in the cranial nerves and descend to include the entire body. The initial neurological signs include double vision, loss of pupillary response to light, drooping eyelids, difficulty eating, slurred speech, and dry mouth. The weakness and paralysis descend to the trunk and extremities and eventually involve respiratory muscles. The mortality rate for foodborne botulism is about 5 to 15%. Death is usually due to respiratory failure.

WOUND BOTULISM

Most cases of wound botulism occur when an anaerobic wound is contaminated with C. botulinum, primarily from the soil. The gastrointestinal signs seen with foodborne botulism are not present, but a patient may develop a fever, and the wound may produce an exudate (pus). Wound botulism resembles foodborne botulism in terms of incubation period and neurological signs.

INFANT BOTULISM

Infant botulism is the most commonly reported form of botulism in the United States and is usually the result of type A or B toxins. It usually affects babies less than 6 months old, although it may also be seen in older infants. Infant botulism results from ingestion of *C. botulinum* spores that grow in the gastrointestinal tract and produce toxins. This differs from foodborne botulism in adults, where the preformed toxin is ingested. The source of the spores is usually unknown, but could include soil, household dust, or vacuum cleaner dust. Some cases have been traced to ingestion of honey that contains the spores. For this reason it is recommended that children under 1 year old should not be given any honey, not even a little bit on a pacifier to sweeten it.

The initial sign of infant botulism, in over 90% of cases, is constipation. This is followed by general weakness, poor feeding with swallowing difficulty, a weak or abnormal cry, and poor head control. Signs of infant botulism can appear as soon as 6 hours following ingestion, and can progress over the next 1 to 4 days. The signs may include progressive muscle weakness that eventually involves respiratory muscles, resulting in respiratory failure. Severity of symptoms will vary, from a mild constipation only to a severe "floppy baby syndrome" to possible death. In some instances the death is so sudden that it is mistakenly reported as sudden infant death syndrome (SIDS). There is no fever associated with infant botulism.

DIAGNOSIS

Diagnosis of botulism in animals is difficult and is often based on ruling out other diseases that present with similar clinical signs. A definitive diagnosis can be made if the toxin is found in the food, feces, vomitus, stomach or intestinal contents, or blood. The toxin is found in blood only in the very early stages of the disease. In the toxicoinfectious form of botulism, in which the animal has acquired the *C. botulinum* organism instead of the toxin, the organism can be cultured from tissue. If the animal has died, stomach or rumen contents and feces should be submitted to a diagnostic laboratory. Feed from the past 2 to 5 days should also be submitted for analysis.

In people, diagnosis of botulism is based on history, clinical signs, and detection of *C. botulinum* or its toxin in feces or serum. Infants with botulism rarely have toxins in the serum, so the feces must be tested. In the case of wound botulism, fluid from the wound is tested for the presence of organisms or toxins. The clinical signs of botulism are not unique to botulism and can be seen in many other diseases. This is why a laboratory must confirm the presence of *C. botulinum* or its toxin to make a correct diagnosis.

Diagnostic tests are performed by state health department laboratories, or by the Centers for Disease Control and Prevention (CDC).

TREATMENT

If botulism is suspected, immediate treatment is essential. Patients with respiratory distress may be put on a respirator for several weeks. Antitoxins are available for types A, B, and E from the CDC, but can be obtained only by a healthcare provider in health departments if botulism is suspected or confirmed. The antitoxin reduces the severity of the disease if it is given early. When treated early enough, most patients recover. Infants with botulism are not given the antitoxin because of the risks involved. Supportive care in a hospital is the only treatment available. Infected wounds must be cleaned thoroughly, usually surgically, to remove the bacteria.

PREVENTION IN ANIMALS

Prevention in animals involves, primarily, good husbandry. Avoid feeding spoiled or contaminated feed, implement rodent control, and properly dispose of dead animals. Do not allow animals to feed on dead animals or decaying carcasses. In some areas where botulism is common, vaccines are available for horses, cattle, sheep, goats, mink, and pheasants.

PREVENTION IN HUMANS

There is no vaccine to prevent botulism in humans. Foodborne botulism can be prevented if proper home-canning methods are used. Wash all foods well before processing them. The U.S. Department of Agriculture (USDA) Extension Service (http://www.uga.edu/nchfp/publications/publications_usda.html) provides current guidelines for processing home-canned meats and vegetables. Local county agents can also usually provide this information.

Before eating home-canned foods, examine the container and the food. A bulging lid or leaking jar indicates food spoilage. Spurting liquid when you open the container, along with an "off" odor and mold, also indicates spoilage. Do not eat these foods. Cook home-canned vegetables and meats before eating them by boiling them for at least 10 minutes. If the foam has an odor, or the food looks spoiled, discard it. Do not discard food where children or animals can eat it.

Honey should not be fed to children under 1 year old because it may contain spores of *C. botulinum*.

All wounds or cuts should be cleaned well and properly bandaged if necessary.

Some unusual and uncommon sources of botulism that have been reported include chopped garlic in oil, chili peppers, tomatoes, and improperly handled baked potatoes wrapped in aluminum foil.

HISTORICAL FACT

Foodborne botulism was first associated with sausage in Europe during the 1880s. There was no refrigeration available to store the meat, which was probably only partially preserved with salt and smoke. Eating bad sausage was associated with the disease that came to be known as botulism, after the Latin word for sausage, *botulus*.

BOVINE SPONGIFORM ENCEPHALOPATHY (MAD COW DISEASE)

Bovine spongiform encephalopathy (BSE), or *mad cow disease*, is a progressive, neurological disorder of cattle. It was first discovered in the United Kingdom in 1986. It has been suggested that BSE is a mutated form of scrapie, seen in sheep and goats, which has been around for centuries. The appearance in cattle may be related to feeding contaminated sheep and/or goat-derived protein supplements to cattle. The word "spongiform" in the name refers to the fact that when an animal dies of BSE its brain is full of holes, like a sponge.

MORBIDITY: +

MORTALITY: ++++

ETIOLOGY: PRION

BSE is caused by a poorly understood protein called a *prion*. When BSE prions are transmitted to humans, the resulting disease is known as *variant Creutzfeldt-Jakob disease* (vCJD). Different prions cause scrapie in sheep and goats, chronic wasting disease in mule deer and elk, feline spongiform encephalopathy, and other neurological diseases in humans.

A prion cannot be classified as bacterial or viral. It is a modified form of a normal component of a cell surface, known as a *prion-related protein*, or *PrP*. Prion diseases, as a group, are also known as *transmissible spongiform encephalopathies* (TSEs) because they cause a variety of diseases, all characterized by progressive, degenerative, neurological disorders that are always fatal.

Prions appear to multiply by converting normal protein molecules into pathogenic ones by inducing the normal molecules to change their shape.

Prion diseases are distinguished by incubation periods measured in years, characteristic spongiform changes in the brain, and lack of an inflammatory response.

TRANSMISSION

Transmission of prions from one animal to another and from animals to humans is not well understood. Evidence points to ingestion of food contaminated with tissues containing the prions. In animal-to-animal transmission, this could happen when an animal is fed protein supplements containing rendered BSE-infected tissues from an infected animal. Tissues that have been found to contain BSE prions are the brain, spinal cord, retina, bone marrow, and distal ileum. People can become infected by eating beef that has been contaminated with BSE prions during slaughter of infected animals and packaging of beef products from these animals.

DISEASE IN CATTLE

After a lengthy incubation period, infected cattle begin to show apprehension, excitability, fixed staring, incoordination, and muscle tremors and fall down. They become hypersensitive to light and touch. Death is inevitable, and most often occurs in less than 2 weeks, although some cases have been known to linger for a year.

DISEASE IN HUMANS

In its progression, vCJD follows a course similar to BSE, affecting predominately younger people. It is associated with depression, coordination problems, mood swings, "pins and needles" or pains in the limbs and feet, bad headaches, cold extremities, rashes, and short-term memory loss. These symptoms worsen over a relatively short time. Death is inevitable, and most often occurs after 6 months. The median duration of vCJD is 14 months.

DIAGNOSIS

There are no clinical, serological, or immunological tests available for diagnosis of BSE or vCJD. Diagnosis is tentatively based on clinical signs and history, and is confirmed by studying a microscopic section of the brain after death. In humans, diagnosis is aided by eliminating other causes of encephalopathies.

TREATMENT

There are no specific treatments for BSE or vCJD. Supportive treatment is given until the patient dies.

PREVENTION

BSE

Cattle should not be fed ruminant-derived protein supplements. Since 1997 the USDA has banned any materials that could be infected with BSE prions from cattle feed. Public health control measures have been instituted in many countries to prevent potentially prion-infected tissues from entering the human food supply. For instance, the United Kingdom excludes all animals more than 30 months old from being used for human food or animal feed supplies.

VCJD

Travelers to countries that have reported cases of BSE can avoid eating beef and beef products. The alternative would be to eat only solid pieces of meat muscle, such as steaks and roasts, which have a lower risk of being infected with BSE prions. Avoid brain or mixed beef products, such as hamburger or sausage, which have a higher risk of being infected with BSE. There is no evidence that milk or milk products transmit BSE prions.

BRUCELLOSIS

Brucellosis, also known as *Bang's disease* in animals and as *undulant fever* or *Malta fever* in humans, can cause abortion in both cattle and humans. The disease has been around a long time. Descriptions of what sounds like brucellosis can be found in the Bible, but the *Brucella* organism was not discovered until 1887, by Sir David Bruce, a Scottish physician. The genus is named after him.

MORBIDITY: +
MORTALITY: + TO +++
ETIOLOGY: BACTERIAL

Brucellosis is caused by bacteria belonging to the genus *Brucella*. They are small, gram-negative coccobacilli. The five species of *Brucella* most commonly associated with brucellosis are *B. abortus, B. ovis, B. suis, B. melitensis*, and *B. canis*. *B. melitensis* is not found in the United States.

HOSTS

Brucellosis has been identified in cattle, sheep, goats, pigs, dogs, horses, bison, elk, reindeer, caribou, many species of deer, camels, foxes, hares, mice, rats, ticks, and fleas. Brucellosis has also been found in seals, otters, and dolphins. Humans can be infected by many of the species of *Brucella*.

B. abortus primarily infects cattle, but is also found in bison, camels, deer, dogs, horses, sheep, and humans.

B. ovis is responsible for testicular inflammation in rams and occasionally for abortion in ewes but does not infect other animals or humans. Goats are susceptible to this species by experimental (deliberate or intentional) infection.

B. suis covers a wider host range than most other *Brucella* species. Pigs, wild hares, reindeer, wild caribou, and rodents are some of the varied hosts of this species.

B. melitensis causes a highly contagious disease in sheep and goats, although cattle can also be infected. *B. melitensis* is the most important species in human infection, but is not found in the United States.

B. canis causes testicular inflammation in the male dog and abortion and uterine infection in the female. It has been reported in no other animal species except humans.

TRANSMISSION

In animals, transmission is by direct contact with an infected animal, or by coming in contact with blood, urine, vaginal discharges, placentas, or aborted fetuses from infected animals. During the period of the *Brucella* life cycle when the bacteria are found in the blood, blood-sucking arthropods may transmit the organism. Domestic and wild canines can spread brucellosis to uninfected herds by dragging dead or aborted fetuses and placentas from the infected herd to the uninfected herd.

Most transmission to humans occurs in one of three ways:
- Drinking unpasteurized milk or eating cheese made from unpasteurized milk, especially soft cheeses. When cattle, sheep, goats, and camels are infected, the *Brucella* organism is found in their milk. Pasteurizing milk will kill the organisms. This is a problem more often for those traveling in countries where there are not effective public health and animal health programs.
- Coming into direct contact with placental tissues or vaginal secretions from infected animals. The *Brucella* organism will most often enter the human body through a wound. This is especially a hazard to people working in the veterinary profession, ranchers, hunters, and people working in slaughterhouses.
- Inhaling an aerosol, which occurs primarily in laboratories where *Brucella* organisms are grown.

Transmission has also been reported through breast milk from an infected mother to her child and through a contaminated tissue transplant. Sexual transmission has also been reported. These cases are extremely rare.

BRUCELLOSIS IN ANIMALS

In animals, brucellosis is usually associated with late-term abortions in females and inflammation in the male reproductive tract.

CATTLE

In cattle, brucellosis is called *Bang's disease*, after Bernhard Lauritz Frederik Bang, a Danish veterinarian, who discovered *B. abortus* as the cause of contagious abortion in cattle in 1887. In cows the organism causes disintegration of the placenta, leading to late-term abortion. In bulls it causes testicular inflammation and sometimes arthritis. Transmission can be through ingestion of the organism or as a sexually transmitted disease (STD). The incubation period can be as short as 2 weeks, or as long as a year or more.

SHEEP AND GOATS

B. melitensis is associated with late-term abortions in sheep and goats or weak lambs or kids. It also causes mastitis, especially in goats. Transmission is through ingestion of the organism. *B. melitensis* is not found in the United States.

  B. suis is a problem in rams, where it causes testicular inflammation. It rarely causes abortion in sheep and goats.

PIGS

B. suis causes abortion at any time during pregnancy in sows, weak or stillborn piglets, and testicular inflammation in boars. Transmission is through ingestion or as an STD.

DOGS

B. canis causes late-term abortion in bitches, early death of puppies, and testicular or scrotal inflammation in stud dogs. Transmission is as an STD. Dogs can become infected with other *Brucella* species if they eat placentas from infected farm animals. Dogs can also develop infection of the spinal discs, leading to back pain and rear leg weakness or paralysis.

CATS

Cats are resistant to *Brucella* infections.

HORSES

B. abortus has been identified as one of the causes of fistulous withers, or poll evil, which results in abscess formation in the area of the withers (the area of the neck between the shoulder blades) or poll (the area behind the ears and just to the rear of the skull). The abscesses may burst and drain on their own, or they may be surgically opened to allow them to drain. The pus from these abscesses contains the *B. abortus* organism and is a source of infection to humans. Infected horses have a history of contact with infected cattle. *B. abortus* has been identified as the cause of late-term abortion in a mare, but this is an unusual occurrence.

BRUCELLOSIS IN HUMANS

Brucellosis in humans is also known as *Malta fever* (because it was first identified on the island of Malta) or *undulant fever* (because of the waves of rising and falling body temperature). The incubation period is usually 1 to 2 months. Some infected people show no clinical signs. In other people, the appearance of clinical signs may be sudden, or they may come on slowly.

Brucellosis first presents with flulike symptoms, such as vomiting, diarrhea, constipation, headaches, chills, weakness, painful muscles, loss of appetite, and weight loss.

In more prolonged cases, patients develop recurrent or undulating fever that spikes in the night (night sweats), extreme fatigue, and arthritis. Men may develop testicular inflammation, and pregnant women could suffer a spontaneous abortion. These signs may last for 2 to 4 weeks, after which the person recovers spontaneously. In other people, the clinical signs seem to appear and disappear in 2- to 14-day intervals. These people can spontaneously recover in 3 to 12 months. Rarely, the disease becomes chronic, with depression, arthritis, and chronic fatigue recurring months after apparent recovery. Death is rare, but when it happens, it is usually associated with an inflammation of the inner lining of the heart (endocarditis).

DIAGNOSIS

ANIMALS

In most animals, serological antibody testing is the most reliable diagnostic test for brucellosis. In the early stages of the disease, the *Brucella* organisms are found in the blood and bone marrow. These fluids may be cultured, but this is not a reliable diagnostic test. Organisms can also be found in the placenta and in the lungs and stomach contents of aborted fetuses.

In pigs, cattle and goats, the tests are done to detect brucellosis in a herd, so not every animal is tested. In sheep it is usually the ram that is tested. In dogs the most reliable diagnostic test is culturing blood, milk, semen, vaginal discharges, aborted fetal tissue, or placenta to isolate *B. canis*.

HUMANS

In humans, an initial diagnosis is based on history and clinical signs. The diagnosis can be confirmed by culturing blood, bone marrow, lymph nodes, cerebral spinal fluid, or abscesses. Serological tests are more commonly used to confirm brucellosis. Cholera, tularemia, *E. coli*, *Salmonella spp.*, and *Pseudomonas spp.* can cause cross-reactions in some serological tests, resulting in a false-positive reaction.

TREATMENT

ANIMALS

There is no effective treatment for brucellosis in most species. Infected animals are removed from the herd. In dogs, infected animals are neutered and no longer used for breeding purposes. In horses, treatment of fistulous withers and poll evil is attempted in some cases. The treatment involves antibiotics and supportive care and is a long process. Extreme care must be taken to prevent human infection from the exudate of the abscesses. For this reason many veterinarians recommend euthanasia of infected horses.

HUMANS
Treatment for brucellosis in humans involves combination antibiotic therapy for up to 6 weeks.

PREVENTION AND CONTROL

ANIMALS
In domestic animals, control is based on identification, segregation, and elimination of infected breeding animals. Since 1951, there has been a joint state and federal cooperative domestic livestock brucellosis eradication program in the United States. It is based on surveillance testing on farms, at stock markets, and at slaughterhouses. Infected animals are traced back to their herd of origin, and the entire herd is quarantined and brucellosis tested. Sometimes entire herds must be destroyed.

Vaccines are available for uninfected herds. The eradication program, along with vaccinations, has nearly eradicated brucellosis in cattle in the United States.

HUMANS
People who travel to countries where brucellosis is prevalent should be careful to not drink unpasteurized milk or eat products made from unpasteurized milk. Hunters should wear rubber gloves when handling the viscera of animals. People who work in veterinary practices, laboratories, stockyards and slaughterhouses should wear protective gear when handling suspect animals, tissues, or fluids. Farmers or ranchers should wear rubber or plastic gloves when assisting calving or aborting animals and should wash and disinfect all potentially contaminated areas when they are finished.

There is no vaccine available for the general public. Immunocompromised people (e.g., cancer patients, HIV-infected individuals, organ transplant patients) should not handle infected dogs.

Brucella organisms can survive up to 6 weeks in dust and up to 10 weeks in soil and water. They are easily killed by common disinfectants and heat, including sunshine.

All cases or suspected cases of brucellosis must be reported to the local health department, who will notify the state health department, Federal Bureau of Investigation (FBI), and local law enforcement. The state health department will notify the CDC.

HISTORICAL NOTE

At one time *Brucella spp.* was considered a possible bioterrorism weapon. In 1999 it was taken off the list of organisms considered likely biologic threats for terrorism, in part because of the long incubation period and the low mortality of infected people. It has since been put back on the list.

CAMPYLOBACTERIOSIS (VIBRIOSIS)
MORBIDITY: +++
MORTALITY: + TO +++
ETIOLOGY: BACTERIAL

There are several zoonotic species of *Campylobacter*, but *C. jejuni* and *C. fetus* are the most pathogenic. *C. jejuni* and *C. fetus* cause two specific diseases in humans and animals, so they will be discussed separately. *Campylobacter spp.* are spiral or curve-shaped, motile, gram-negative rods. The genus *Campylobacter* was previously known as *Vibrio*.

CAMPYLOBACTER JEJUNI

C. jejuni causes gastroenteritis (stomach and intestinal inflammation).

HOSTS

Mammals, the intestinal tracts of birds, and raw poultry meat are the primary reservoirs of the bacteria.

TRANSMISSION

Most human cases of campylobacteriosis are transmitted through handling raw poultry or eating raw or undercooked poultry meat. Poultry meat becomes infected when birds are slaughtered and feces from the intestines contaminate the meat. Cross-contamination of other foods can occur in the kitchen if the raw poultry or poultry juices come in contact with other food. *Campylobacter* can also be transmitted by direct exposure to infected animal feces. Animals that shed *C. jejuni* in their feces don't have to be clinically sick to pass the bacteria to humans. Person-to-person infection is possible, especially in adults caring for children with voluminous diarrhea. People with compromised immune systems (from HIV, organ transplants, or cancer treatment) are more susceptible to *Campylobacter* infection and its complications.

C. jejuni can also be transmitted through drinking raw or unpasteurized milk or feces-contaminated water.

Animals are infected most often by eating feces-contaminated food, undercooked poultry, and drinking feces-contaminated water. Infected children may transmit the disease to puppies and kittens, which can in turn infect others.

CAMPYLOBACTER JEJUNI IN ANIMALS

Young animals are more susceptible to campylobacteriosis.

DOGS AND CATS

The clinical signs are more severe in puppies and kittens and include vomiting and diarrhea. Pet owners can become infected by coming in contact with contaminated feces.

CATTLE

Calves infected with *C. jejuni* may show clinical signs, including fever and diarrhea with blood or mucus present. The disease can last up to 2 weeks. *C. jejuni* has been shown to cause mastitis in cows, which can be a source of infection to humans and animals who drink the raw milk.

SHEEP

C. jejuni causes abortion in sheep, which will occur late in pregnancy. An infected ewe may deliver a full-term lamb that will be dead or weak and that may die within a couple of days.

POULTRY

Poultry are reservoirs for *C. jejuni*, and shed the organism in their feces. They do not naturally become clinically ill.

CAMPYLOBACTER JEJUNI IN HUMANS

Campylobacteriosis is one of the most common diarrheal diseases in the United States and is seen most often in the summer months. Clinical signs appear 2 to 5 days after exposure and include nausea, vomiting, watery diarrhea, bloody diarrhea, abdominal cramping, and fever.

Guillain-Barré syndrome, a nervous system disorder that can lead to paralysis when the body is triggered to attack its own nerves, is a rare complication of *C. jejuni* infection. It will appear about 2 weeks after the appearance of clinical signs and will last several weeks.

DIAGNOSIS

Diagnosis is based on serology (checking the serum for the presence of antibodies against the *C. jejuni* organism). Multiple samples must be tested to follow the level of antibodies as the disease progresses. Many apparently healthy animals shed *C. jejuni* in their feces, so culturing the feces is not diagnostic.

TREATMENT

Most cases of campylobacteriosis are self-limiting and do not require any specific treatment. Keeping the patient hydrated when diarrhea is present is important. In some cases, antibiotics may be necessary to decrease the severity of the disease, especially if there is a high risk of human exposure.

CONTROL

Campylobacteriosis is difficult to control in animals because of widespread reservoirs in wild animals. In humans, strict personal hygiene when in contact with people or animals with diarrhea is essential. Avoiding raw milk, contaminated drinking water, undercooked or raw poultry meat, and cross-contamination of other foods will also decrease the chance of becoming infected. Freezing reduces the number of *C. jejuni* organisms on meat.

CAMPYLOBACTER FETUS

C. fetus causes vibriosis, also known as *bovine venereal campylobacteriosis*, or *BVC*. The disease is characterized by infertility, fetal death, and abortion.

HOSTS

Cattle and sheep are hosts. Humans are rarely infected.

TRANSMISSION

This is an STD in cattle. Infections are spread by infected carrier bulls to susceptible cows during mating.

In sheep the transmission is oral, from ingestion of aborted fetuses, placentas, or vaginal discharges.

In humans transmission is not well understood. It may involve ingestion of contaminated food or water, transplacental infection, or other contact with infected animals.

CAMPYLOBACTER FETUS IN ANIMALS

Infertility, early embryonic death, and abortions result from *C. fetus* infections.

CATTLE

In cows, *C. fetus* causes endometritis (inflammation of the lining of the uterus) and salpingitis (inflammation of the fallopian tubes) that can last 3 to 4 months. A cow becomes infected when she is bred with an infected bull. Most bulls are asymptomatic and recover spontaneously due to natural immunity. Some bulls carry the organism for years and can be an unsuspected source of infection.

An infected cow will come back into heat after she is bred, indicating she is not pregnant. This can happen repeatedly. Of infected cows that eventually become pregnant, 5 to 10% will abort between 4 and 8 months. Other infected cows will eventually recover and have a normal pregnancy. Some cows will retain the organism and pass it back to the bull during the next breeding cycle. After an infection, cows can become naturally immune to further infection. Some cows will not develop sufficient natural immunity and may become infected again.

C. fetus can also be transmitted by contaminated equipment and instruments used in artificial insemination.

SHEEP

C. fetus, along with *C. jejuni*, causes fetal death and abortion during late pregnancy. Full-term lambs may be born dead or so weak that they die within a couple of days. Ewes can develop endometritis and septicemia (bacterial infection in the blood), which can be fatal. Ewes develop natural immunity after infection that may last up to 3 years. In some ewes, the bacteria can locate in the gall bladder and be shed in feces. Because transmission is oral, this is not an STD in sheep.

CAMPYLOBACTER FETUS IN HUMANS

In humans, *C. fetus* appears to be an opportunistic organism that usually manifests itself in people who are already ill. It rarely causes enteritis comparable to that caused by *C. jejuni*.

In men, *C. fetus* causes septicemia that usually occurs as a secondary infection to an already existing primary infection. If septicemia develops, the mortality rate can reach over 40%.

In pregnant women, the clinical signs are seen after the fifth month of pregnancy and include fever, diarrhea, miscarriage, or premature births. Premature and full-term babies can die from the infection, which is characterized by inflammation of the central nervous system. The mortality rate in babies is 50%.

DIAGNOSIS

Diagnosis is initially based on a herd history of infertility and abortion. *C. fetus* organisms are very fragile and are quickly destroyed by heating, drying, and exposure to the atmosphere. Without preservation in special media, they must be cultured within a couple of hours of collection. For this reason culture is not a reliable diagnostic test. Antibodies against *C. fetus* may be detected in vaginal mucus from females, washings from the prepuce of males, and tissue from aborted fetuses. These tests must be done in a diagnostic laboratory.

In men with septicemia, the *C. fetus* organism is usually an unsuspected finding when the blood is cultured. When central nervous system (CNS) signs (headache, back pain, fever, weakness, sensory loss, stiff neck, nausea, paralysis, seizures, coma, or disorientation) are present, the organism can be found in the cerebral spinal fluid. Culturing the organism from vaginal fluid is difficult and requires repeated cultures in special media.

TREATMENT

Antibiotics can be infused into the uterus of females and the sheath of males. Most animals recover spontaneously. Finding animals to treat can be difficult because many animals show no physical signs of disease.

CONTROL

Vaccines are available for cattle and sheep and must be administered before the breeding season.

Artificial insemination will eliminate the spread of *C. fetus* from the bull to cows. Equipment and instruments must be cleaned between each use to prevent infection from infected cow to uninfected cow through contamination.

Because of oral transmission in sheep, control also involves good sanitation, such as prompt removal of aborted fetuses and placentas. Ewes that have aborted should be isolated from the rest of the herd. Some ewes will shed *C. fetus* in their feces and contaminate grazing areas. Clothing and tools that are contaminated with *C. fetus* can also be a source of infection.

CAT SCRATCH DISEASE

Cat scratch disease (CSD) is also called *cat scratch fever*. It is also known as *regional lymphadenopathy*, or *lymphadenitis*. Even though the disease has been described since 1889, the causative agent was not positively identified until 1992.

MORBIDITY: ++
MORTALITY: +
ETIOLOGY: BACTERIAL

CSD is caused by *Bartonella henselae*, a small, gram-negative rod. The disease is seen worldwide and is most commonly diagnosed during the fall and winter months, possibly because this is when cats spend more time indoors.

HOSTS

Cats are the primary reservoir of *B. henselae* for human infection.

TRANSMISSION

B. henselae is transmitted from cats, primarily kittens less than 1 year old, to humans by a bite, lick, or scratch. There are a number of theories about how cats are originally infected. One theory suggests that the cat is a mechanical vector for the organism that is spread from cat to cat by fleas. The organism in the flea feces is picked up in the cat's mouth when it bathes and is distributed to the cat's feet during subsequent baths. The incidence of CSD decreases when the presence of fleas is controlled. CSD is seen more commonly in warmer climates, where the number of fleas is greater than in cooler climates.

Another theory states that *B. henselae* may be part of the normal flora in a cat's mouth that is spread to the cat's feet when it bathes.

B. henselae is found in an infected kitten's bloodstream on a recurring, cyclical basis that may be short-lived or can last for months or years. *B. henselae* can be transmitted from one cat to another through blood transfusion, but not transplacentally from mother to kittens, and not sexually.

CSD is not contagious from human to human or from human to cat. Fleas have not been implicated in the spread of CSD directly to humans. A person with CSD does not have to be isolated from the rest of the family.

CAT SCRATCH DISEASE IN CATS

Cats rarely get clinically ill from *B. henselae* infection. Many adult cats have antibodies to *B. henselae* in their blood, indicating a previous exposure to the organism.

CAT SCRATCH DISEASE IN HUMANS

CSD in humans is usually self-limiting, without any permanent damage. Most cases are seen in people under 21 and those in the veterinary profession. There is usually, but not always, a history of a cat scratch or bite. Letting a cat lick an open wound can also result in CSD. A small pustule resembling an insect bite develops at the site within 3 to 10 days (Figure 5). In 1 to 2 weeks, lymph nodes near the area will become swollen and painful (lymphadenopathy). Nearly half of the people who develop the pustule will also develop a headache, mild fever, and lethargy. The lymph nodes of the neck and extremities are most often affected because most cat bites and scratches occur on the arms and legs. The lymphadenopathy is unilateral, on the side where the infection occurred. Nearly a quarter of infected patients will develop very painful,

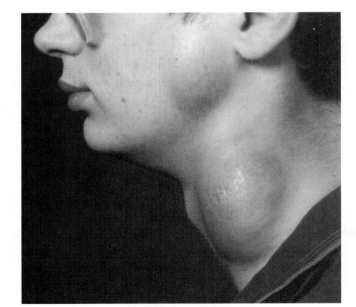

FIGURE 5.   Enlarged lymph nodes in a person with cat scratch disease. (From Greene CE: *Infectious diseases of the dog and cat*, ed 3, St Louis, 2006, Saunders.)

pus-filled lymph nodes (lymphadenitis). Even though CSD is self-limiting, it can take up to 3 weeks for the lesion at the site of infection to heal and several months for the lymph nodes to return to their normal size. In mild cases, treatment is usually not required.

Some atypical consequences of CSD have been seen in people who are not in good health, or people with compromised immune systems. These include *bacillary angiomatosis*, which results in many blood-filled cysts on the skin, and *Parinaud's oculoglandular syndrome*, which resembles pink eye (conjunctivitis). Only one eye may be involved and shows signs that include a soft granuloma (polyp) developing on the palpebral conjunctiva (the mucous membrane lining the inner surface of the eyelid). The lymph nodes in front of the ear become swollen and painful. The patient usually does not recall being scratched or bitten by a cat. It is possible that the organism is found in cat saliva that stays on the fur after a cat bathes. The patient becomes infected after petting the cat, then rubbing the eye, thus transmitting the organism from the fur to the conjunctiva.

Another atypical condition, seen less frequently, is encephalitis (inflammation of the brain) resulting in seizures.

These abnormal signs and syndromes are also self-limiting, although it may take up to a year for them to resolve.

DIAGNOSIS

CATS

Diagnosis of *B. henselae* infection in cats can be difficult. Five tests are available, but none is better than the others.

- Enzyme-linked immunosorbent assay (ELISA), immunofluorescence assay (IFA), and Western blot tests detect the presence of antibodies against *B. henselae* in blood. A positive test indicates that the cat has been exposed to *B. henselae* at some time during its life. It does not indicate an active infection. It has been shown that over 10% of the *B. henselae* organisms in blood will not stimulate antibody production, so these cats will test negative even though there are organisms present.
- Blood culture would be the ideal method of detection if the organism stayed in the blood 100% of the time, rather than appearing and disappearing on a repeating, cyclical basis. A positive culture would provide a definitive diagnosis because the organisms themselves were in the blood when the sample was taken for culture. A negative culture would indicate only that the organism was not present in the blood when the sample was taken.

- Polymerase chain reaction (PCR) detects the presence of *B. henselae* DNA in the blood, but the same drawback exists for PCR as for blood culture. PCR will detect the DNA only if the organism is circulating in the blood at the time the sample is taken.

HUMANS

Most cases of CSD in humans are based on clinical signs, along with a history of a cat bite or scratch. The same tests used to diagnose *B. henselae* infection in cats can be used for confirmation of the diagnosis in humans.

TREATMENT

Cats rarely show clinical signs of illness due to *B. henselae* infection, so treatment is rarely implemented. A 3-week regimen of specific antibiotic treatment may rid the cat of the organism and eliminate the cat as a source of infection. This is not done on a routine basis.

Human cases of CSD usually resolve themselves without treatment. In more severe cases, treatment with an antibiotic may shorten the course of the disease. Symptomatic treatment of fever and pain with over-the-counter medications will reduce discomfort but will not affect the course of the disease. The atypical manifestations of CSD are most often treated with antibiotics, though the patient will most likely recover without treatment.

PREVENTION AND CONTROL

One episode of CSD usually results in lifetime immunity from further infections. The following are some guidelines for decreasing exposure to CSD:
- Keep cats indoors.
- Avoid playing rough with kittens who like to bite and scratch when they play.
- Scrub cat bites and scratches immediately with warm water and soap. Apply hydrogen peroxide to the wound after scrubbing.
- If you have open wounds on your hands and arms, wear gloves when handling cats.
- Do not allow a cat to lick an open wound.
- Keep the cat's claws trimmed. Declawing is not necessary.
- Control fleas with approved flea-control products.
- Teach people not to pick up strange cats.
- Routinely wash hands after handling or playing with cats.

IMMUNOCOMPROMISED PEOPLE AND CAT SCRATCH DISEASE

Immunocompromised people may develop more severe, but usually not life-threatening, cases of CSD, so some precautions should be taken. They should adopt only adult (older than 1 year), indoor cats from a known source, rather than pick up a stray cat or kitten. Kittens are more likely to be infected with *B. henselae*. A cat with suspected *B. henselae* infection does not have to be given to another home or euthanized if proper precautions are taken as previously described.

HISTORICAL NOTE

"Cat Scratch Fever" is also a song, written and performed by Ted Nugent.

COLIBACILLOSIS

Colibacillosis is a disease caused by the bacterium *Escherichia coli*. Colibacillosis is also known as *hemorrhagic colitis*. Other names associated with colibacillosis are *colibacteriosis*, *colitoxemia*, and *enteropathogenic diarrhea*. We will concentrate on *E. coli* O157:H7, which has emerged as a significant cause of food poisoning in people.

MORBIDITY: ++
MORTALITY: + TO ++
ETIOLOGY: BACTERIAL

Colibacillosis is caused by *E. coli*, which is a facultative anaerobic (can grow both aerobically and anaerobically), gram-negative, rod-shaped bacterium that ferments sugar, which results in gas production. The gas is released from the body as flatulence. *E. coli* is one of several bacteria normally found in the intestines of humans and animals.

There are hundreds of strains of *E. coli*. Most of the strains are essential for normal food digestion and do not cause disease as long as they stay in the intestinal tract. Some of the normally nonpathogenic *E. coli* will become pathogenic in other organs. For example, if *E. coli* from the intestines gets into the urinary system, it can cause cystitis. In fact, *E. coli* is the primary cause of cystitis.

The strains that cause intestinal diseases are grouped into six categories. The three most important categories are enterotoxogenic *E. coli* (ETEC), enteroinvasive *E. coli* (EIEC), and enterohemorrhagic *E. coli* (EHEC).

The ETEC strains produce toxins that cause profuse watery diarrhea, abdominal cramping, dehydration, and possibly vomiting. The EIEC strains invade intestinal lining cells and cause a mucoid diarrhea that may become tinged with blood.

The EHEC strains are the most zoonotic and pathogenic strains. They attach to intestinal wall cells and produce strong toxins. *E. coli* O157:H7 is the strain that has emerged as a significant cause of food poisoning in people. When *E. coli* O157:H7 enters the intestinal tract of a person, it produces a powerful toxin that damages the wall of the intestines, resulting in bloody diarrhea.

HOSTS

The most common reservoir of *E. coli* O157:H7 is cattle. Other animals that have been identified as sources of human infection are deer, swine, and (rarely) dogs and horses. None of these animals gets sick from harboring *E. coli* O157:H7.

When *E. coli* O157:H7 enters the intestinal tract of a human it becomes pathogenic and may cause severe disease. The organism is passed in human feces and is infective to other people.

TRANSMISSION

Transmission of *E. coli* O157:H7 is by the fecal-oral route. *E. coli* O157:H7 is passed in the feces of infected animals, primarily cattle. When people put anything in their mouths that has been in contact with the infected feces, they may become infected. An infected person can also infect other people (Figure 6).

The most common method of transmission is eating undercooked, contaminated ground beef. Meat can be contaminated with feces on its surface

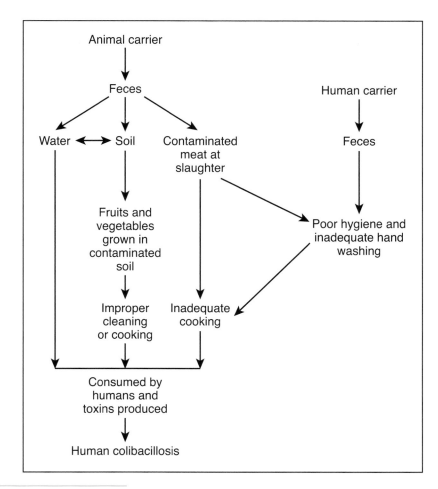

FIGURE 6.   Colibacillosis.

during the slaughtering process. When ground beef is made, the surface *E. coli* O157:H7 is mixed throughout the meat. Infected meat looks and smells normal, but must be adequately cooked to kill the *E. coli* O157:H7. Other cuts of meat, such as roasts, may be contaminated only on the surface, but must also be adequately cooked to kill the organism. Salami and sausage that might contain infected ground beef will also become infective if not cured or cooked properly.

Water can become contaminated when infected feces are washed into lakes, rivers, ponds, streams, or municipal water sources. Drinking this untreated water can lead to illness. Increased contamination is often seen after heavy rain showers, when feces are washed into the water source, or in the spring, when melted snow runoff enters the water.

Alfalfa sprouts, spinach, radish sprouts, and lettuce have been sources of infection. Any raw fruit or vegetable has the potential to be infected with *E. coli* O157:H7 if it comes in contact with infected feces. This is especially true if it is grown in soil fertilized with raw cattle manure or irrigated with contaminated water.

If infected feces get on the udder of a dairy cow, the *E. coli* O157:H7 organism may contaminate the milk from that cow. The raw milk will be infective, so it must be pasteurized to kill the organism. The same is true for dairy products made from the infected milk.

Improperly processed apple cider and apple juice have been identified as sources of infection. Any fruit juice must be pasteurized to kill the *E. coli* O157:H7 organism.

Person-to-person transmission occurs when good sanitation procedures are not followed. Not washing hands with warm soapy water after using the toilet, changing diapers, or handling raw meat has led to transmission of *E. coli* O157:H7 to other people.

COLIBACILLOSIS IN ANIMALS

Animals, especially cattle that harbor *E. coli* O157:H7, do not get sick.

Other strains of *E. coli* have been associated with calf scours (diarrhea), mastitis, abortion and early foal death in horses, neonatal enteritis in newborn pigs, gut edema in older suckling pigs, and inflammation of numerous tissues and organs in poultry.

COLIBACILLOSIS IN HUMANS

Some people who are infected with *E. coli* O157:H7 do not get sick. Others will typically start showing clinical signs within 3 to 9 days. Abdominal cramping and pain is followed in about a day with diarrhea. Initially the diarrhea will be watery, but then becomes bloody. Patients sometimes vomit, but rarely have a fever. People who are otherwise healthy will recover without treatment in 5 to 10 days.

Some people, especially children under 5 years old and adults over 65 years old, may develop one of two serious complications to *E. coli* O157:H7 infection:

- Hemolytic uremic syndrome (HUS) is characterized by destruction of red blood cells, kidney failure, decreased platelet formation, and some neurological signs. Renal failure is the predominant symptom. HUS is the principal cause of kidney failure in young children in the United States. HUS can be followed with long-term complications, and it can be fatal in 3% to 5% of cases.
- Thrombotic thrombocytopenic purpura (TTP) is characterized by the same symptoms as HUS, only the neurological signs, such as seizures, strokes, and coma, predominate. This syndrome is seen most often in elderly people and can be fatal up to 50% of the time.

DIAGNOSIS

Diagnosis of *E. coli* O157:H7 is based on finding the bacterium in feces by culturing the feces in a special medium. This medium is not normally used to culture *E. coli*, so it has to be specially requested. Any person developing sudden watery or bloody diarrhea should be tested for *E. coli* O157:H7.

TREATMENT

Most people who develop only diarrhea will recover without specific treatment, which would include antibiotics, in 5 to 10 days.

Treatment for HUS and TTP includes dialysis, transfusions, and supportive care.

PREVENTION

Prevention of *E. coli* O157:H7 infection is based on good sanitation procedures and common sense:

- Cook all ground beef to a core temperature of at least 160° F.
- Keep raw meat away from foods that will be eaten raw. Wash counters, utensils, and hands in warm soapy water after working with raw meat.
- Drink only pasteurized milk, fruit juices, and apple cider. Most commercially available products have been pasteurized.

- Wash all food that will be eaten raw.
- Drink only safe water. Municipal water systems treat water for *E. coli* using chlorine, ozone, or ultraviolet light. When camping, treat water by boiling or filtering before brushing teeth, washing dishes, or making beverages such as coffee or tea.
- People with diarrhea should avoid public swimming places. They should also avoid sharing baths and preparing food for others.
- Avoid swallowing swimming pool or other water where people are swimming.
- If children are allowed to touch animals, especially cattle, at farms, petting zoos, or fairs, make sure they wash their hands with warm, soapy water afterward. Watch children to make sure they do not put dirty hands in their mouths.
- People with diarrhea, especially children, must wash their hands with warm, soapy water following every bowel movement and every time they change a diaper.

CRYPTOSPORIDIOSIS (CRYPTO)

Cryptosporidiosis is one of the most common forms of waterborne diarrhea in the United States. Although it has been a veterinary problem for quite a while, it was not identified in humans until 1976.

MORBIDITY: +++
MORTALITY: +
ETIOLOGY: PARASITIC

Cryptosporidiosis is caused by a microscopic, one-celled, protozoan parasite, *Cryptosporidium spp.*

HOSTS

Cryptosporidium spp. can infect mammals, reptiles, fish, and birds. *C. parvum* is the species that most often infects humans, pets, and domestic and wild animals.

TRANSMISSION

Cryptosporidiosis is spread by the fecal-oral route. This means people or animals can get cryptosporidiosis when they put anything in their mouths that has been in contact with the feces of an infected animal or human. The most common sources of infection are direct contact with infected feces, water contaminated with infected feces (human or animal), and food contaminated by infected feces (Figure 7).

Infective organisms called *oocysts* are passed in the feces of an infected host. Oocysts have thick, protective outer shells and can live in a moist environment for up to 6 months. When the oocysts are ingested by the next host, they lose their thick outer shells and enter the epithelial cells of the gastrointestinal tract of the host. In these cells, they undergo an asexual multiplication and a sexual multiplication, which result in oocyst production. The oocysts leave the cells and are passed in the feces.

A second, uncommon route of transmission is through the respiratory tract. In this instance the oocysts become airborne on feces, such as when a calf with diarrhea swishes its tail or when a high-pressure washer is used to clean up feces. When this method of transmission occurs, respiratory signs, along with intestinal signs, may result.

Transmission does not occur through contact with blood.

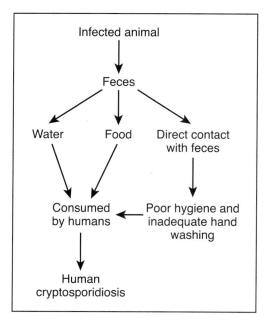

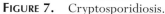
FIGURE 7. Cryptosporidiosis.

CRYPTOSPORIDIOSIS IN ANIMALS

Cryptosporidiosis in animals affects mainly very young animals or immuno-compromised animals. Calves 1 to 3 weeks old and lambs appear to be the most susceptible. Pigs, horses, dogs, and cats can become infected, but infection is uncommon in these species.

Clinical signs of cryptosporidiosis appear after a 4-day incubation period. They are characterized by profuse, watery diarrhea; lack of appetite; straining to defecate when there are no feces to pass; and weight loss. Cryptosporidiosis may be worse in immunocompromised animals.

Some animals may be infected without exhibiting any clinical signs. These animals will still shed oocysts and will be a source of infection to other animals.

Cryptosporidiosis is self-limiting in otherwise healthy animals. Mortality is very low in animals that develop cryptosporidiosis. Neonates and immunocom-promised animals will have a longer course of disease that is increasingly fatal.

CRYPTOSPORIDIOSIS IN HUMANS

Anyone can get cryptosporidiosis. In humans, as in animals, cryptosporidiosis affects primarily young children and immunocompromised people, such as those receiving chemotherapy, kidney dialysis, or steroid therapy, and people with HIV/AIDS or Crohn's disease. Cryptosporidiosis may linger longer and may, in some cases, be fatal in these people. Dehydration is a common sequel to diarrhea. Pregnant women are more susceptible to dehydration when they have cryptosporidiosis.

The clinical signs of cryptosporidiosis in humans appear after a 2- to 7-day incubation period. They include watery diarrhea, nausea with or without vomiting, abdominal cramping (especially on the right side), mild fever, loss of appetite, and headache. The disease is self-limiting in 1 to 2 weeks in otherwise healthy people. During that time, the signs may come and go in a cyclical manner.

Some people will be infected with *Cryptosporidium spp.* and show no clinical signs. These people can be a source of infection for other people or animals.

Although anyone can get cryptosporidiosis, there are certain groups of people who are at increased risk of becoming infected:

- Veterinarians and veterinary technicians who work around young animals, especially calves and lambs
- Dairy farmers, cattle ranchers, and their families
- People who are immunocompromised
- People exposed to human feces during sexual contact
- Children in childcare facilities who come in contact with diaper-age children
- People who work in childcare facilities
- Parents of infected children
- Caregivers working with people with diarrhea
- People who go camping, hiking, or backpacking and drink contaminated water from lakes, streams, rivers, ponds, or shallow wells
- People who swallow water from swimming pools, lakes, rivers, or ponds contaminated with infected feces

DIAGNOSIS

Cryptosporidiosis is diagnosed by identifying oocysts in fecal samples. Sometimes multiple samples will have to be analyzed to find the oocysts because they are so small and may be shed in cycles.

TREATMENT

There is no specific treatment for cryptosporidiosis in otherwise healthy people at this time, although there is a drug that has been approved for use in people with healthy immune systems. Supportive therapy, mainly to prevent dehydration, is given to patients exhibiting clinical signs.

Cryptosporidium is resistant to many disinfectants. It can survive in an adequately chlorinated swimming pool for several days. Moist heat (65° C for 30 minutes), steam, freezing, or thorough drying are the best ways to destroy oocysts on utensils or other objects that may have been contaminated.

PREVENTION

There are no vaccines available for protection against cryptosporidiosis. Prevention of cryptosporidiosis is based on good hygiene.

ANIMALS
- Raise animals, especially newborns, in a clean, dry environment.
- Separate healthy animals from sick animals. Caretakers should take care of the healthy animals first or have a separate caretaker for sick animals.
- Rotate areas where animals are confined so there is a time when their cages can be cleaned and disinfected.
- Clean up feces every day. The oocysts are infective when they are passed in the feces.

PEOPLE
- Wear gloves when working around animals with diarrhea, especially young animals. If there is a danger of being hit in the face with feces, as with a swishing tail, wear a surgical mask or face shield.
- Wash hands thoroughly with warm water and soap after working with any animal with diarrhea, even if gloves were worn.
- Do not eat or drink in an animal facility. Wash hands before eating or drinking after working with animals.
- Wash hands thoroughly with warm water and soap after using the toilet, before handling food, or after changing diapers.
- Do not let diapered children with diarrhea go swimming.
- Clean all surfaces that may come in contact with feces, such as bathroom fixtures, diaper pails, changing tables, and toys (human and animal).
- Do not drink untreated water from lakes, ponds, streams, rivers, swimming pools, shallow wells, hot tubs, or Jacuzzis. Water can be treated by boiling it for 2 to 3 minutes, or by using a filter with a pore size of no bigger than 1 micron that has been rated for cyst removal.
- Wash in safe water and/or peel all fruits and vegetables before eating them.

- Use safe water to wash dishes, brush teeth, and make ice cubes.
- Do not eat or drink unpasteurized dairy products; they may have been contaminated with feces.
- Be especially careful when traveling to developing countries. Cryptosporidiosis is found worldwide.
- Avoid fecal exposure during sexual activity, especially anal-oral activity. The cases of reported cryptosporidiosis rose dramatically in the early 1980s, along with the HIV/AIDS epidemic.

DERMATOMYCOSIS

A dermatomycosis is a highly contagious skin disease caused by fungi. It affects both people and animals. Other names for a dermatomycosis are *tinea*, *ringworm*, *jock itch*, and *athlete's foot*. There are three groups of fungi that can cause dermatomycosis:

- Anthrophilic fungi use humans as their primary reservoir.
- Geophilic fungi live in the soil and cause ringworm in people and animals.
- Zoophilic fungi live on animals other than people, but can be transferred to people.

    We will deal only with zoophilic fungi that are transmitted from animals to people.

MORBIDITY: +

MORTALITY: +

ETIOLOGY: FUNGAL

Two genera of zoophilic fungi, *Microsporum* and *Trichophyton*, are responsible for nearly all cases of dermatomycosis that are zoonotic. The spores of these fungi are able to survive in the environment, in protected areas, for 18 months or more. They rely on keratin, a protein found in the outer layer of the skin, hair, feathers, nails, and hooves, for survival. They thrive when on a person or animal, on shed hair, or on dead skin cells.

HOSTS

Dermatomycosis in animals is called *ringworm*. Cats, dogs, cows, horses, sheep, and rodents are the most common sources of zoonotic dermatomycoses. The following zoophilic fungi are responsible:

- *Microsporum canis* is carried by cats and dogs and causes the most common form of ringworm in these animals. It is transmissible to people (Figures 8 and 9).
- *Trichophyton mentagrophytes* causes ringworm in rodents, cats, dogs, horses, cattle, and pigs. It is transmissible to people (Figure 10).
- *Trichophyton equinum* is found on horses and rarely on people (Figure 11).
- *Trichophyton verrucosum* is carried primarily by cattle, but can be found on people, horses, and sheep (Figures 12 and 13).
- *Microsporum nanum* causes ringworm in pigs. It is rarely found on people.

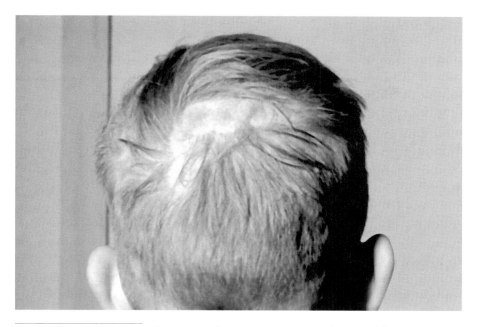

FIGURE 8. *Microsporum* infection in a human. (Courtesy Public Health Image Library, PHIL 3968, Centers for Disease Control and Prevention, Atlanta, 1959.)

TRANSMISSION

Not every person or animal that comes in contact with these fungi will develop clinical disease. Some animals and people will be carriers while remaining asymptomatic. Young animals and children are most often affected because their immune systems are not fully developed. The same is true for people with suppressed immune systems, such as people with HIV/AIDS, those receiving chemotherapy, and organ transplant recipients.

Animal dermatomycosis is transmitted by direct contact with an infected animal or with items contaminated with fungal spores. Grooming equipment, brushes, blankets, bedding, tack, carpeting, furniture, air filters, shed hair, or any other item that comes in contact with an infected animal can become contaminated with spores. Spores can survive in a boarding facility or any place an infected animal has visited, including veterinary facilities.

The incubation period varies in animals and people but is usually a few days to a few weeks.

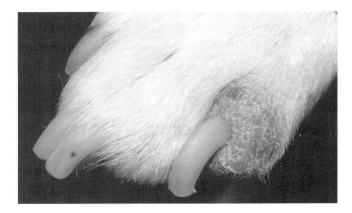

FIGURE 9.   *Microsporum canis* in a cat: the alopecia and erythema of the lateral digit are typical of nail bed infections caused by *M. canis*. (From Medleau L, Hnilica KA: Small animal dermatology: a color atlas and therapeutic guide, ed 2, St Louis, 2006, Saunders.)

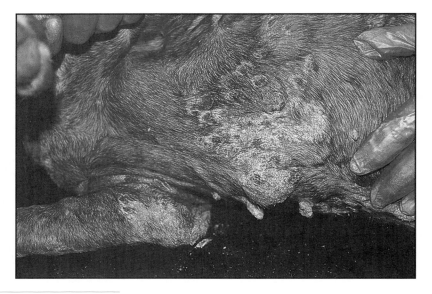

FIGURE 10.   *Trichophyton* infection in a dog. (Photograph by Annette Loeffler, with permission. From Gaudiano F, Curtis C: *Veterinary dermatology: a manual for nurses and technicians,* London, 2005, Elsevier.)

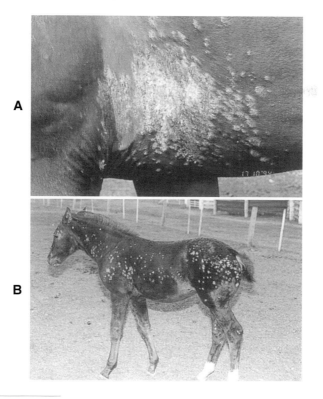

FIGURE 11.   *Trichophyton* infection in a horse. **A**, Ringworm: diffuse infection with *Trichophyton* in the girth and chest wall areas due to infection from contaminated girths and riding boots. **B**, Ringworm: generalized infection with *Trichophyton* in a 6-month-old foal. (From Pascoe RRR, Knottenbelt DC: *Manual of equine dermatology*, London, 1999, Saunders.)

DERMATOMYCOSIS IN ANIMALS

Many animals carrying the fungal spores that cause ringworm will show no clinical signs. Young animals are most likely to develop ringworm lesions.

The lesions typically seen with ringworm usually begin with scaly patches containing broken hairs. The areas may become inflamed and turn red, swollen, and crusty. In some animals the lesions are not well-defined and may be more diffuse. In these cases, the animal shows areas of alopecia that may become ulcerated if the animal licks or scratches the site. Itching is not a common problem with ringworm.

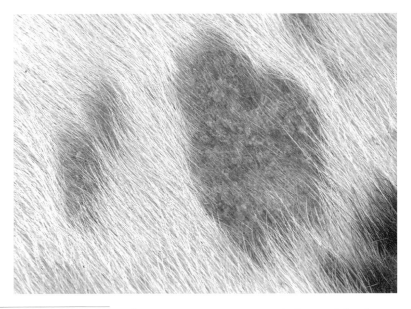

FIGURE 12.   *Trichophyton* infection in a cow. Note irregularly ovoid, hairless areas with mild surface crusting. (Courtesy Dr. H. Denny Liggitt. From McGavin MD, Zachary JF: *Pathologic basis of veterinary disease,* ed 4, St Louis, 2006, Mosby.)

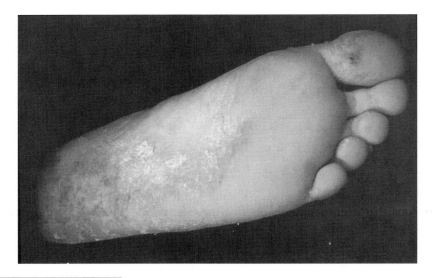

FIGURE 13.   *Trichophyton* infection in a human. (Courtesy Public Health Image Library, PHIL 2938, Centers for Disease Control and Prevention, Atlanta, 1964.)

CATS AND DOGS

M. canis is the most common cause of ringworm in cats and dogs. *T. mentagrophytes* is a less common cause. Other geophilic fungi can also cause ringworm. Kittens are most likely to show clinical signs. Lesions are found on the face, ears, and paws. Nearly 90% of infected, asymptomatic cats carry *M. canis*. Most people who develop ringworm will do so from contact with infected cats or kittens. Dogs usually develop the typical circular lesions associated with ringworm. The lesions can be found anywhere on the body and initially look like shaved areas. Pustules may develop in the lesions.

RODENTS AND LAGOMORPHS

Most rodents and rabbits will develop ringworm from *T. mentagrophytes* infection. The lesions are white and scabby and are seen on the head and trunk. *T. mentagrophytes* is transmissible to dogs and cats as well as people. Most rodents are asymptomatic carriers.

HORSES

Ringworm lesions caused by *T. equinum* are found mainly where saddles and harnesses rub the skin. It is also known as *girth itch*. The lesions appear as exudative patches, where the hair sticks together because of the sticky pus present on the skin. When these clumps fall off or are pulled away, they leave behind areas of alopecia. The skin becomes thickened. Itching is a problem only in the initial stages. Transmission to people occurs but is rare.

CATTLE

Ringworm in cattle, also known as *barn itch*, is caused by *T. verrucosum*. In range cattle, it is seen during the winter months, when cattle are more likely to come in contact with one another because they are confined to barns or feedlots. The lesions are seen mainly on the face (especially around the eyes, ears, and muzzle) and neck but also appear on the flanks and legs. They are white, dry areas containing broken hairs. Initially the lesions may look like warts. Some lesions are very small (1 centimeter), and others are quite extensive. A scab develops that eventually falls off, leaving behind an area of alopecia. Cattle ringworm is transmissible to people.

SHEEP AND GOATS

Ringworm is rare in goats. A condition known as *club lamb fungus* has been recognized since the late 1980s. This is a form of ringworm that develops in sheep, mainly lambs, that are taken to shows, exhibitions, sales rings, or any place lambs from different herds are brought together. It has also been known as *woolrot* and *lumpy wool*. *Trichophyton* has been identified as the causative fungus. Close shearing, repeated washings, and stress make the lambs more susceptible to infection. The lesions appear on the head, neck, and back. They initially appear as thick, red, oozing, circular areas that later become crusty. The wool may appear clumped, and hairs at the center of the lesion break off easily. Transmission to people can occur.

PIGS

M. nanum is classified by some as a geophilic fungus because it is found in soil where pigs are raised and is seldom spread to people. The lesions in pigs are wrinkled areas of skin covered by a thin scab that is easily removed.

DERMATOMYCOSIS IN HUMANS

It is important to remember that animals are a minor source of dermato-mycosis in people. In healthy people, lesions stay on the keratinized layers of skin and hairs, but in people with suppressed immune systems, the infection can go deeper and become systemic. Fungal skin infections in people are named by where they are found on the body:

* *Tinea corporis* is seen on the skin. The lesions appear as small, red spots that grow into large rings on the arms, legs, or chest.
* *Tinea pedis* is also known as *athlete's foot*. The lesions usually begin between the toes, where the skin is moist. They become red and itchy and have a wet surface. If the fungus spreads to the toenails, it becomes *tinea unguium*. The toenails become thick and crumbly. Scratching the area can spread the infection to hands and fingernails.
* *Tinea cruris*, also known as *jock itch*, is caused by fungus growing in the moist, warm area of the groin. The lesions are found most often in men who frequently wear athletic equipment.
* *Tinea capitis*, also known as *ringworm*, is found on the head. The lesions begin as itchy, red areas where eventually the hair is destroyed, leaving bald patches. Ringworm is the most common dermatomycosis in children.

DIAGNOSIS

Beyond the clinical signs, there are three methods used to diagnose dermatomycosis:

* The Woods lamp is a special blacklight that emits filtered ultraviolet light. When exposed to a Woods lamp, many but not all fungi will fluoresce bright blue-green. A lack of fluorescence does not indicate that no fungus is present. Dander and certain topical medications will also fluoresce.

- Hair is pulled from the outer edges of the lesion, where the fungi are still active. The hairs are placed on a microscope slide in a KOH (potassium hydroxide) solution to make the spores more visible. They are then examined under a microscope for the presence of spores on the hair shaft. This method of diagnosis is useful up to 70% of the time.
- For identification of the specific fungus causing the dermatomycosis, hair from the edge of the lesion must be cultured on specialized media in a specific environment. Growth can take up to several weeks, and each fungus grows in uniquely appearing colonies on the media.

TREATMENT

Most cases of dermatomycosis resolve spontaneously in time, as immunity inhibits the lesions from spreading, but medical treatment can lessen the severity of the disease and decrease the possibility of it spreading to other animals or people. Both topical and oral medications are available, some of them over the counter. Topical medications include creams, ointments, sprays, shampoos, and dips. Anyone who has had to suffer the smell of lime sulphur dip for treatment of ringworm in a cattery knows that prevention is much better than treatment. Treatment may last a long time, even after the animal or person appears better. The fungus can remain even after the hair has grown back.

PREVENTION

There is only one vaccine available in North America against ringworm in cats caused by *M. canis*. No other vaccines are available for people or other animals. Prevention is based on limiting exposure to infected animals or people and anything with which they might have come in contact. This is difficult because the fungal spores can survive in the right environment for up to 18 months or longer. Some precautions that will help limit the exposure of people to infected animals follow:

- Screen new animals introduced into a herd or colony.
- Begin treatment immediately on any animal that develops lesions.
- Maintain hygienic living conditions for animals. Reduce crowding as much as possible to avoid direct contact.
- Open sores, scratches, and other skin lesions may enhance the development of ringworm in an animal, so minimize exposure to any sharp object that may cause injury.
- When infected animals are present, clean all bedding, toys, tack, carpeting, furniture, kennels, stalls, barns, or anywhere the animal has been. The spores

are killed by sunlight, a 1:10 household bleach solution (1 part bleach to 10 parts water), and strong detergents. Vacuuming will remove the spores, but remember to destroy the vacuum bag afterward.

- Disinfect all grooming equipment after each use. Commercial fungicides are available for this purpose.
- Be cautious when taking animals to fairs, shows, boarding kennels, grooming facilities, and veterinary facilities. Look for animals with obvious lesions and avoid them and the places they inhabit.
- Healthy, well-nourished animals and people are more resistant to dermato-mycosis.
- Since fungi prefer moist areas for growth, keep kennels, barns, and other living quarters as dry as possible.
- Wear gloves when handling potentially or obviously infected animals.

EASTERN EQUINE ENCEPHALITIS
MORBIDITY: +
MORTALITY: +++
ETIOLOGY: VIRAL

Eastern equine encephalitis virus (EEEV) is an arbovirus (*arthropod-borne virus*) that causes eastern equine encephalitis (EEE). Other important encephalitis arboviruses include the western equine encephalitis virus, St. Louis encephalitis virus, West Nile virus, and La Crosse encephalitis virus.

HOSTS

Hosts are vertebrates, especially birds, humans, and horses.

TRANSMISSION

EEEV is seen primarily east of the Mississippi River. The natural hosts for EEEV are passerine birds, such as blackbirds, finches, jays, sparrows, and warblers. The virus is found mainly in or near swampy areas or wetlands and is transmitted through the bite of an infected mosquito. Horses and humans are infected when a mosquito takes blood from an infected bird and subsequently takes blood from a horse or human and deposits the virus at the site of the bite. Horses and humans do not develop a significant enough *viremia*, or virus level in the blood, to be a source of infection to other animals via a mosquito bite; they are, therefore, considered dead-end hosts (Figure 14).

　　EEE is *indirectly zoonotic*, meaning humans and horses cannot be infected directly, from one another, or from birds. Mosquitoes act as vectors that transmit the virus. EEE occurs most commonly during late summer and coincides with mosquito activity.

EASTERN EQUINE ENCEPHALITIS IN HORSES

EEEV in horses causes a central nervous system (CNS) disease. An infected horse either dies suddenly or shows progressive signs of CNS deterioration, with death 2 to 3 days after the onset of clinical signs. Mortality can reach 75% to 90% in infected animals. Mildly infected horses may recover over a 2-week

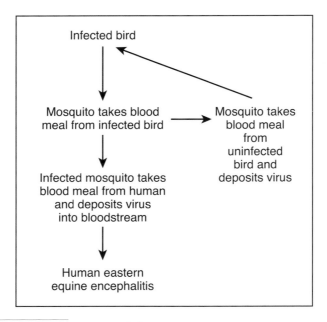

FIGURE 14.   Eastern equine encephalitis.

period but are left with some degree of permanent brain damage. All equines (e.g., mules and donkeys) are susceptible to EEEV infection. Birds such as ostriches, emus, quails, turkeys, and pheasants are also susceptible to EEEV infection.

The first clinical sign of EEE is a fever, seen a day after infection and lasting a day. This sign is often overlooked. The second phase of clinical signs is seen 4 to 6 days after infection and includes a second episode of fever; depression; anorexia with difficulty swallowing; flaccid lips; teeth grinding; staggering gait; stumbling; walking in circles; paddling when down; a "sawhorse" stance with splayed, stiff legs; head pressing; sensitivity to light; blindness; convulsions; paralysis; and death. The course of EEE in horses is shorter (5 to 10 days) and the mortality rate is higher than with western equine encephalitis or West Nile encephalitis.

EASTERN EQUINE ENCEPHALITIS IN HUMANS

In humans, EEE first presents with flulike symptoms, somewhere between 4 and 15 days after being bitten by an infected mosquito. These symptoms include fever, vomiting, fatigue, headaches, neck stiffness, and generalized muscle pain. In some people, the symptoms will progress to seizures and possibly coma. If CNS signs develop, mortality can reach 35%. If a person recovers from an EEEV infection that has progressed to CNS signs, there is about a 30% chance that permanent brain damage will remain. EEE is seen less often than western equine encephalitis or St. Louis encephalitis, but it causes a more severe disease with a higher mortality rate.

DIAGNOSIS

A specific diagnosis is made by isolating EEEV from the brain tissue of humans or horses who have died from EEE. An initial diagnosis is based on clinical signs, season, and geographic location. A final diagnosis can be made by virus isolation or by serologic testing of the affected patient for the presence of antibodies against EEEV.

TREATMENT

There is no specific antiviral drug treatment for EEE. Supportive therapy such as administration of medications to decrease brain swelling, nutritive fluids, and antibiotics to treat or prevent secondary bacterial infections may make the patient more comfortable.

PREVENTION

HORSES
Prevention of EEE in horses involves vaccination and decreased exposure to mosquitoes. There is no evidence that EEE can be transmitted directly between horses, between humans, or between horses and humans.

Reducing exposure to mosquitoes involves the following steps:
• Drain areas of standing water. These are mosquito breeding sites.
• Keep horses inside during peak mosquito activity (early evening until after dawn).
• Keep the lights off in stables during the night. Mosquitoes are attracted to incandescent lights.
• Put screens on stable windows and keep fans blowing to prevent mosquito access.
• Place incandescent lights around the outside of the stable, to attract the mosquitoes away from the horses.
• Fog the stable with an approved pesticide in the evening.

- Use mosquito repellents intended specifically for horses.

Vaccines are available for protection against EEEV infection and should be administered either before mosquito season begins in colder climates or when a foal reaches 3 months of age in areas where mosquito activity is nearly constant. Initial vaccination requires multiple injections followed by yearly boosters.

HUMANS

Prevention of EEE in humans involves decreased exposure to mosquitoes. There is no vaccine available.

Reducing exposure to mosquitoes involves the following steps:
- Drain areas of standing water. These are mosquito breeding sites.
- Reduce outdoor activities during peak mosquito activity.
- Wear protective clothing when mosquitoes are most active, especially in the early evening and early morning. Protective clothing includes light-colored, long-sleeved shirts and long pants.
- Use insect repellent containing DEET on exposed skin.
- Make sure window screens fit properly and do not have any holes to decrease mosquito access to building interiors.

EHRLICHIOSIS

Ehrlichiosis is a group of tick-borne diseases that attack white blood cells. It is a seasonal disease that corresponds to the months when ticks are active. In dogs the disease is also known as *tracker dog disease*, *canine hemorrhagic fever*, or *canine typhus*.

MORBIDITY: +
MORTALITY: +
ETIOLOGY: BACTERIAL

Ehrlichia spp. are small, gram-negative, obligate intracellular coccobacilli that cause ehrlichiosis. There are many species that cause disease in various animals, but the zoonotic species are *E. chaffeensis*, *E. ewingii*, *Anaplasma phagocytophilum* (formerly *E. equi* and *E. phagocytophila*), and *Neorickettsia sennetsu* (formerly *E. risticii*). *E. canis* may be zoonotic, but confirmation has not been completed. *Ehrlichia* bacteria must infect white blood cells to multiply. Within the cells, they multiply to form large aggregates called *morulae*, which are visible on a stained blood smear. The white blood cells are responsible for protection of the body from outside invaders, so damage to these cells and their consequent removal from circulation can make the host more susceptible to developing diseases.

HOST

The host for ehrlichiosis depends on the species of *Ehrlichia*.

TRANSMISSION

Ixodid (hard) ticks are vectors for ehrlichiosis. The Lone Star tick is the primary vector for *E. chaffeensis* and *E. ewingii*. *A. phagocytophilum* is transmitted by black-legged ticks. The vector for *N. sennetsu* is unknown. The organisms are transmitted from host to host by tick feedings. Ticks at all stages of the tick life cycle (Appendix 1) can become infected when they feed on an infected host (Figure 15).

Rarely, ehrlichiosis has been transmitted via blood transfusions. Direct person-to-person or person-to-animal transmission does not occur.

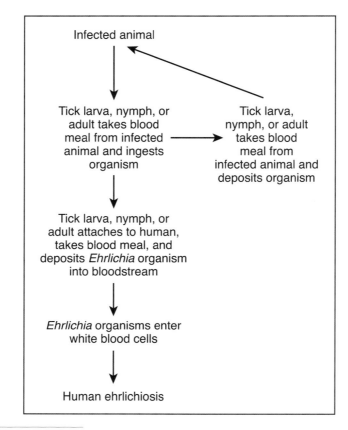

FIGURE 15.   Ehrlichiosis.

EHRLICHIOSIS IN ANIMALS

E. chaffeensis has been identified in dogs, coyotes, red foxes, deer, goats, and lemurs. The primary reservoir hosts are deer. *E. ewingii* causes disease in dogs; dogs are also the primary reservoir hosts. *Anaplasma phagocytophilum* is found in dogs, horses, deer, bison, elk, rodents, llamas, cats, cattle, sheep, goats, and nonhuman primates. The primary reservoir hosts are deer, elk, and rodents. *Neorickettsia sennetsu* is still a mystery. It causes a mild disease.

Ehrlichiosis in animals is named by which white blood cells are infected. *Monocytic ehrlichiosis* is characterized by infection of monocytes and macrophages. If granulocytic white blood cells, primarily neutrophils, are infected, then the disease is *granulocytic ehrlichiosis*.

DOGS

Monocytic ehrlichiosis and granulocytic ehrlichiosis present similar clinical diseases. The incubation period for monocytic ehrlichiosis is 8 to 20 days; for granulocytic ehrlichiosis, it is 1 to 14 days after a tick bite. Dogs usually present with fever, lethargy, anorexia, swollen lymph nodes, enlarged spleen, and weight loss. They may also develop vomiting, diarrhea, lameness, edema in the hind legs, coughing, difficulty breathing, and discharges from the eyes and nose. The acute phase lasts up to 4 weeks, and many times dogs will recover spontaneously. Some dogs recover clinically but still harbor the bacteria to develop a subclinical disease. During the subclinical phase a dog may remain symptom-free, clear the bacteria from its body, or develop chronic ehrlichiosis. Chronic ehrlichiosis is characterized by anorexia; chronic weight loss; fever; depression; weakness; edema in the hind limbs, scrotum, and tail; bleeding disorders; pale mucous membranes; nose bleeds; blood in the urine; or blood in the feces. Many of these signs are attributable to decreased numbers of not only white blood cells but also red blood cells and platelets. Polyarthritis is seen more often in dogs with granulocytic ehrlichiosis than with monocytic ehrlichiosis.

HORSES

Equine granulocytic ehrlichiosis can progress from a mild disease to a severe disease over several days. The initial signs include fever and anorexia progressing to incoordination, depression, jaundice, reluctance to move, and edema of the hind limbs.

CATTLE AND SHEEP

Tick-borne fever in sheep and cattle is caused by *A. phagocytophilum*. Young lambs born in tick-infested areas or introduced to older animals are usually more often infected than older sheep. A sudden fever that lasts 4 to 10 days can be accompanied by weight loss, lethargy, coughing, and increased respiratory and heart rates. In older animals abortion may occur, and the quality of semen may be reduced.

Dairy cattle recently turned out to pasture are most commonly affected by tick-borne fever. The clinical signs include depression, anorexia, decreased milk production, coughing, abortions, and decreased semen quality. Abortion accompanied by decreased milk production and respiratory disease are the two most common syndromes seen.

Most ruminants recover spontaneously within 2 weeks, but relapses brought on by stress can occur. Infections can last up to 2 years after initial recovery.

EHRLICHIOSIS IN HUMANS

Ehrlichiosis in people can be divided into two categories, depending on which white blood cells are infected. If the monocytes and macrophages are infected, it is called *human monocytic ehrlichiosis (HME)*. When the granulocytic white blood cells are infected, it is called *human granulocytic ehrlichiosis (HGE)*. The clinical signs of HME and HGE are virtually the same. Because human ehrlichiosis and Rocky Mountain spotted fever (RMSF) have the same geographic distribution, the same tick vector, and present very similar clinical pictures, ehrlichiosis has sometimes been referred to as *spotless Rocky Mountain spotted fever*. The rash associated with RMSF is rarely seen with ehrlichiosis.

Ehrlichiosis in people varies, from asymptomatic to a nonspecific disease to a potentially fatal disease. The usual incubation period is 5 to 14 days, but symptoms may not appear for up to a month. It starts with flulike symptoms including fever, chills, headache, muscle pain, nausea, vomiting, diarrhea, joint pain, and abdominal pain. Rarely a rash may develop in children, but not as specific a rash as seen with Lyme disease, which may be associated with a very specific appearing rash. The rash usually involves the trunk, legs, arm, and face but spares the hands and feet.

More severe clinical signs, seen more often in immunocompromised people and those who have had their spleens removed, include prolonged fever; kidney failure; secondary infections; heart disease; multiorgan failure; and central nervous system involvement, including seizures and coma. The spleen is one of the organs that filters blood to remove abnormal blood cells. If the spleen is removed, many of the infected white blood cells stay in circulation. In some cases ehrlichiosis can be confused with infectious mononucleosis, which is characterized by fever, lethargy, anorexia, swollen lymph nodes, and enlarged liver and spleen.

DIAGNOSIS

Initial diagnosis is based on patient history of a tick bite, clinical signs, and laboratory tests. Serologic testing will confirm the disease. Morulae are occasionally found in the white blood cells on a stained blood smear (Figure 16).

TREATMENT

Antibiotics are used in the treatment of ehrlichiosis. Early treatment will result in better results; if treatment is not started right away, the course of the disease as well as the treatment may be more prolonged.

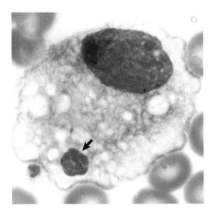

FIGURE 16.   *Ehrlichia* organisms in a white blood cell. (From Harvey JW: Atlas of veterinary hematology: blood and bone marrow of domestic animals, St Louis, 2001, Saunders.)

PREVENTION

Tick and rodent control are the best approach to prevention. Avoiding endemic regions during the peak transmission months is especially important for people who have had their spleens removed or for immunocompromised persons.

Decrease exposure to ticks by following these guidelines:
- Avoid areas where ticks thrive as much as possible. Ticks have to live where their hosts live, so areas that are endemic for specific ticks are where specific species of *Ehrlichia* will be found.
- Wear light-colored clothing when entering an area that may be a habitat for ticks. This will make the ticks easier to see and remove before they become attached.
- Wear long-sleeved shirts and long pants tucked into socks so the ticks cannot crawl under clothing; wear high rubber boots and a hat for the same reason.
- Walk in the center of trails to avoid vegetation where ticks are lurking. Ticks cannot fly, jump, skip, or hop, so they must come in direct contact with a host before they can attach themselves. Immature ticks are found hiding in the shade in a moist area. Adult ticks cling to grass, bushes, and shrubs and wait for a host to come by.
- Exposed skin and clothing can be protected with insect repellents containing DEET. Clothes, but not exposed skin, can be protected with insect repellents containing permethrin, which kills ticks on contact.
- Check often for ticks while outside. Black-legged ticks are tiny and easy to miss.
- Do not sit on the ground or on stone walls, where ticks can abound.

- Make daily checks of the entire body for ticks. Look especially in areas where ticks like to attach, such as behind the ears, the back of the neck, in the armpits, behind the knees, and in the groin area. Bathing will remove crawling ticks but will not detach ticks already attached. Daily tick checks and prompt removal of attached ticks are vital to reducing the risk of transmission. Removing a tick within 24 hours of attachment will greatly reduce the possibility of *Ehrlichia* transmission.
- Wash and dry outdoor clothing in hot temperatures after use.

To remove a tick, use fine tweezers, grasp the tick as close to the skin as possible, and pull straight back with a slow, steady force. Avoid crushing the tick's body. Kill the tick by dropping it in alcohol. Save the tick in alcohol as a possible diagnostic aid.

Tick-control products such as tick collars should be used on dogs that could possibly be exposed to ticks. This will help protect them from possible *Ehrlichia* infection and will help decrease the number of ticks the dogs could possibly bring into a house, where people could be exposed to them.

Grazing ruminants on relatively tick-free pastures will reduce the number of cases of tick-borne fever.

There are no vaccines available to protect against ehrlichiosis.

NOTE

Co-infection with *Borrelia burgdorferi* (Lyme disease), *Babesia sp.,* or other organisms that share the same tick vectors may also be seen.

GIARDIASIS *(GIARDIA)*

Giardiasis is the second most common cause of parasitic human diarrhea in America. The most common cause is pinworms, which are not zoonotic. *Giardia* is the most common cause of water-borne disease. Giardiasis is found in all regions of the United States and has been called *back-packer's disease*, *beaver disease*, and *traveler's diarrhea*.

MORBIDITY: ++

MORTALITY: +

ETIOLOGY: PARASITIC

Giardiasis is caused by a microscopic, single-celled, protozoan parasite, *G. intestinalis,* also known as *G. lamblia.* There have been other *Giardia* species identified, but *G. intestinalis* is considered the primary cause of giardiasis in humans and warm-blooded animals.

G. intestinalis has a two-stage life cycle. In the first stage, the disease-causing trophozoite stage, *G. intestinalis* is found in the small intestine. In the second stage, the cyst stage, the organism is passed in the host's feces. At this stage, it can remain viable in a moist environment for several months because of its thick protective capsule. The cysts can even withstand short-term freezing. Cysts present in the environment are swallowed when a potential host eats feces-contaminated food, drinks feces-contaminated water, or puts any feces-contaminated object in its mouth. The protective capsule is removed by the acid in the stomach, and two trophozoites are formed. The trophozoites are carried to the first part of the small intestine, where they attach to the intestinal wall and reproduce by binary fission. Some of the trophozoites will encyst and pass in the feces. Some unencysted trophozoites will also pass in the feces (Figure 17).

HOSTS

Giardiasis is found in humans and a wide variety of domestic and wild animals including dogs, cats, cattle, sheep, horses, pigs, guinea pigs, chinchillas, deer, mice, beavers, bears, and muskrats. Theoretically, any warm-blooded animal, domestic or wild, could be susceptible.

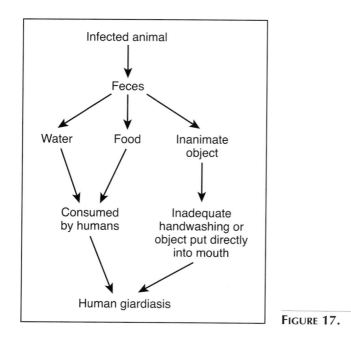

FIGURE 17. Giardiasis.

TRANSMISSION

Giardiasis is spread by the fecal-oral route and can be very contagious. The host must ingest feces contaminated with *G. intestinalis* cysts via food, water, hands, or an inanimate object. When the cysts are passed in the feces of an infected host they are immediately infective, and it takes very few ingested cysts to cause infection.

Outbreaks of giardiasis have been seen where municipal water treatment plants have failed to filter *G. intestinalis* out of contaminated water.

Transmission can be from person to person, animal to animal, person to animal, or animal to person. *Giardia* is not transmitted through blood.

GIARDIASIS IN ANIMALS AND HUMANS

Giardiasis is the same in animals and humans. The disease is more often seen in young animals and children, probably because they are more apt to put contaminated items in their mouths.

The symptoms of giardiasis appear 7 to 10 days after ingestion of the cysts. They include severe, foul-smelling diarrhea; nausea; abdominal cramps; gas; fatigue; and weight loss in the presence of a normal appetite and normal food intake. There is usually no fever and no blood in the diarrhea; feces are usually formed, not watery, and are mixed with mucus. The symptoms usually last about 2 weeks but may last as long 2 months or even as long as a year. Some cases are fatal. In young animals, growth may be retarded.

Some people are exposed to giardiasis more than others. They include people who work with animals, those living in crowded living conditions with poor sanitation, people who work in child care facilities, young children in child care facilities, people exposed to human feces by sexual contact, people who travel to developing countries, and people who spend time in the wilderness and drink untreated water from streams or lakes.

People and animals who are immunocompromised may develop more severe symptoms when infected with *G. intestinalis*.

The mechanism by which *G. intestinalis* causes disease is not known. Not all people or animals who are infected with *G. intestinalis* will develop symptoms of disease. They can, however, be a source of infection to others.

DIAGNOSIS

Diagnosis of giardiasis is based on finding cysts or, less frequently, trophozoites in fecal samples. Because the cysts and trophozoites are shed intermittently, it is necessary to examine a series of at least three fecal samples. A history of recent travel to developing countries, hiking, camping, and drinking untreated water from streams or lakes can be helpful in establishing a diagnosis.

Serologic tests have been developed to detect the presence of *Giardia* antigens in blood.

TREATMENT

Giardiasis is treated with appropriate antibiotics. Some people and animals recover without treatment. Bathing an infected animal and disinfecting the animal's environment with a quaternary ammonium–based disinfectant is also recommended.

PREVENTION

Prevention of giardiasis is based on good sanitation practices to prevent ingestion of any feces-contaminated food, water, or object.

The following recommendations will help campers and hikers prevent giardiasis:
• Make sure the water you drink is safe. Many state parks will post "boil water" warnings. If in doubt, boil water for 3 to 5 minutes. Bottled water is

safe if it has been processed through reverse osmosis. For camping, there are filters available that will remove *Giardia;* read the label to make sure. Chemical purification will also destroy *Giardia*.

- Do not make ice cubes from untreated water.
- Use treated water when brushing teeth, rinsing food that will not be cooked, washing dishes, and making coffee or baby formula.
- Avoid drinking water that may be contaminated with animal or human feces.
- Dispose of waste materials in such a way that they cannot contaminate surface or ground water.

   The following recommendations will help everyone practice good sanitation:

- Wash your hands with soap and safe water after using the toilet, changing diapers, gardening, handling animals, or dealing with animal feces.
- Do not drink unpasteurized milk or eat unpasteurized dairy products; they may have been contaminated with feces.
- Do not go into swimming pools, hot tubs, Jacuzzis, fountains, rivers, springs, ponds, lakes, or streams if you have diarrhea. Avoid swallowing any water from any of these sources.
- Do not prepare food for others if you have diarrhea.
- Teach children how to wash their hands after using the toilet or handling animals.
- Wash all foods to be eaten raw with safe water.
- Wash surfaces that may have come in contact with feces, such as changing tables, diaper pails, bathroom fixtures, dog toys, kennels, pens, or any other animal housing facility.
- Do not drink untreated water during a municipal outbreak.

   Vaccines are available for dogs and cats.

HANTAVIRUS PULMONARY SYNDROME

Hantavirus pulmonary syndrome (HPS) was first identified in the United States in 1993, though it has probably been around a lot longer. It is characterized by a severe lung disease for which there is no cure.

MORBIDITY: +
MORTALITY: +++
ETIOLOGY: VIRAL

The virus that causes HPS belongs to a group of viruses of the genus *Hantavirus*. There are many hantaviruses, and each species has a specific rodent or group of rodents as its main reservoir. In Europe and Asia, *Hantavirus* causes hemorrhagic fever with renal syndrome and is usually not fatal. In North America, *Hantavirus* attacks the respiratory system causing HPS, which has a nearly 50% fatality rate.

HOSTS

Four rodents that have been identified as reservoirs for the HPS virus are the deer mouse, found throughout North America; the cotton rat, found primarily in the southeastern United States, in areas overgrown with shrubs and tall grasses; the rice rat, found in marshy and semiaquatic areas of the southeastern United States; and the white-footed mouse, found in all of the United States except New England. These animals prefer brushy and wooded areas but can be found in more open areas. The deer mouse was the first rodent identified as a reservoir.

Common house mice and common rats have not been associated with HPS.

TRANSMISSION

The most common method of HPS virus transmission to humans is when people breathe air that contains aerosolized, fresh rodent urine, feces, or saliva (Figure 18). Aerosolization occurs when dust or nesting materials are stirred up and tiny droplets containing the virus become airborne. Other methods of transmission that have been identified or suspected are direct transfer, as when a rodent bites a person, or indirect transfer, as when people touch something that has been contaminated with infected rodent excrement and

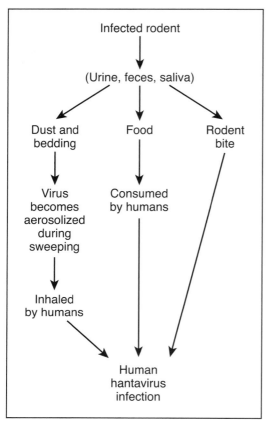

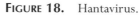

FIGURE 18.   Hantavirus.

then touch their noses or mouths or when people eat food contaminated by rodent excrement.

Transmission occurs anywhere there is an active rodent population. Some of the more common places are homes, summer cottages that have been shut up all winter, barns, sheds, warehouses, storage facilities, restaurants, office buildings, garages, crawl spaces, and vacant buildings. Campers and hikers can become infected if they stay in rodent-infested shelters or pitch tents in rodent-infested habitats.

HANTAVIRUS PULMONARY SYNDROME IN ANIMALS

HPS is not a problem in animals. Rodents carrying *Hantavirus* do not get sick. Pets, domestic animals, and wild animals have not been identified as victims of HPS.

HANTAVIRUS PULMONARY SYNDROME IN HUMANS

HPS is a rare disease. Since its discovery in 1993, fewer than 400 cases have been reported. Not all people who are exposed to *Hantavirus* get sick. For those who do get sick, HPS starts with flulike symptoms that progress to respiratory failure, which can lead to death. Unlike many other diseases that primarily attack people with weakened immune systems, HPS seems to attack healthy people. The incubation period has not been determined, but it appears to be between 1 and 5 weeks. Initial symptoms include fever, fatigue, muscle aches, headaches, dizziness, chills, nausea, vomiting, diarrhea, and abdominal pain. These symptoms are not specific to HPS and may be mistaken for the flu. The patient begins coughing and experiencing shortness of breath as the lungs fill with fluid, 4 to 10 days after the early signs appear. This happens because the virus damages the capillary walls in the lungs, allowing fluid to enter air spaces. If no supportive therapy is provided, a patient may suffocate from the fluid in the lungs.

DIAGNOSIS

Early symptoms are not specific to HPS, so it is often only when the patient starts experiencing respiratory distress that HPS is considered. Serologic tests are available for the detection of antibodies in infected people. A history of exposure to rodent urine, feces, or saliva is helpful.

TREATMENT

There is no treatment for HPS. Suspected patients are placed in intensive care and put on respirators to help them breathe. The longer the time between the appearance of symptoms and the placement of the patient in intensive care, the more likely HPS will be fatal. HPS will be self-limiting if the patient can be kept alive long enough.

PREVENTION

There is no vaccine to protect against HPS. Prevention is based on eliminating or decreasing exposure to fresh rodent urine, feces, and saliva. The virus can live only a few days in the environment, so there has to be an active rodent infestation. Signs of active infestation include:
• Wild rodents in the house. Rodents are more active at night.

- Rodent droppings. Look under sinks, where food is stored, in cupboards, on beams, in old furniture, inside boxes, and in drawers.
- Rodent nests. They will be in protected areas, near food and water sources. They will be found in the types of areas where droppings are found.
- Boxes, containers, and foods that appear nibbled.
- Rodent feeding stations, where there is more evidence of excrement, plus areas where leftover food trash, such as paper, plastic, or cockroach carcasses, accumulates.
- Evidence of gnawing on wood or other hard materials. Rodent teeth grow continuously, so rodents must gnaw on hard surfaces to keep them short.
- Closed rooms with a stale, musty smell.

If rodents are found, they must be eliminated. If no rodents are found, they must be prevented from entering the area. Some of the ways to do this follow:

- Keep houses clean. Do not let foods, including pet food, sit around uncovered. Dispose of garbage in containers with tight-fitting lids. Wash dishes, counters, and floors. Set covered bait station traps or spring-loaded traps if you suspect rodents are in the house. Traps can also be set outside. Make sure pets and children cannot come in contact with traps.
- Seal all holes larger than $1/4$ inch in diameter in screens or walls. Seal both inside and outside walls. Look for and seal gaps under doors, around vents and pipe openings, around fireplaces, around windows and doors, behind appliances, and under kitchen and bathroom sinks.
- Keep areas around houses and other buildings free of brush, overgrown grass, and junk. This will help eliminate nesting areas.
- Put metal flashing around the base of wooden, adobe, or earthen buildings. The flashing should go 12 inches up from the ground and be set 6 inches under ground.
- Elevate feed, hay, woodpiles, and garbage cans at least 12 inches off the ground.
- Spray any rodent feces, rodent nests, dead rodents, or materials that look like they have been infested with rodents with disinfectant before handling them. Commercial disinfectants will work if they are labeled as disinfectants. A homemade disinfectant solution (1.5 cups of household bleach to 1 gallon of water) can be used instead of a commercial disinfectant.
- Wear a respirator, gloves, overalls, and boots when sweeping out buildings that show any evidence of rodent infestation. Spray the area with a disinfectant before and after sweeping.
- When cleaning a building that has been closed for a while and is infested with rodents, let the building air out for at least 30 minutes before cleaning it. Stay out of the building while it is airing out.

HOOKWORMS

Hookworms belong to the phylum *Nematoda*, which contains worms that are round and unsegmented. Members of this phylum are called *nematodes*. There are thousands of species of nematodes, but only seven are of zoonotic importance in North America. These are *Ancylostoma braziliense*, *A. caninum*, *A. tubaeformis*, *Uncineria stenocephala*, *Toxocara canis*, *Toxocara cati*, and *Baylisascaris procyonis*.

    T. canis, *T. cati*, and *B. procyonis* are nematode parasites that are discussed under roundworms.

MORBIDITY: +

MORTALITY: +

ETIOLOGY: PARASITIC

A. braziliense, *A. caninum, A. tubaeformis*, and *U. stenocephala* are all capable of infecting dogs and cats. When the immature larvae of these parasites are found in atypical or dead-end hosts, a disease called *cutaneous larva migrans (CLM)* or *creeping eruption* develops. The most severe cases of CLM are associated with *A. braziliense* infection.

HOSTS

A. braziliense is the hookworm of dogs and cats, seen primarily in the southeastern United States. *A. caninum* is the most common hookworm of dogs in tropical and subtropical areas, *A. tubaeformis* is the most common hookworm of cats in tropical and subtropical areas, and *U. stenocephala* is the hookworm of dogs and cats in cooler regions of the United States and Canada. Humans are considered atypical or dead-end hosts.

TRANSMISSION

Adult hookworms are found attached to the wall of the small intestine. They feed on the host's blood. During the normal life cycle of hookworms, eggs are passed by adult females in dog or cat feces and hatch as larvae on the ground. In 1 to 3 weeks they become infective larvae. The infective larvae are found in shady, moist, sandy soil. The larvae infect the host either by being ingested or by penetrating the host's skin (Figure 19).

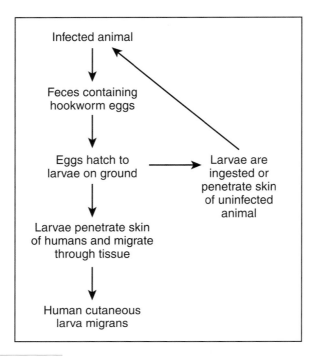

FIGURE 19.   Cutaneous larva migrans.

Larvae that enter the host through minute breaks in the skin migrate to the lungs via the bloodstream. Once in the lungs, they break out of the blood vessels and enter the alveoli, then crawl up the respiratory tree to the trachea, where they cause a mild irritation that makes the host cough. Coughing brings the larvae to the mouth, where they are swallowed and travel to the small intestine, attach to the wall, and mature to adulthood.

If the larvae are ingested, they travel directly to the small intestine. Some of the larvae stay there, and some burrow through the intestinal wall and travel to the lungs through tissues. Once in the lungs, they follow the same path as larvae that penetrated the skin. Some of the larvae that are traveling through tissue encyst and stay in the tissue, until the (female) host becomes pregnant. Near the end of the pregnancy, these encysted larvae become active, and either finish their migration to the lung and on to the intestines, or they travel to the mammary glands, where they congregate and are passed in the milk to the newborn offspring.

If the infective larvae accidentally penetrate the skin of a human through minute breaks, they are unable to penetrate any further than the outer layer of the skin. They cannot penetrate into blood vessels and travel to the lung. Humans are considered atypical or dead-end hosts. Many people are infected by walking barefooted on beaches, where dogs and cats have been allowed to roam freely and contaminate the sand with infected feces.

HOOKWORMS IN ANIMALS

In dogs and cats, adult hookworms attach to the small intestine and suck blood. Heavy infections can lead to severe anemia and sudden death, especially in young puppies and kittens and in animals that are weak or malnourished. Milder infections can manifest as anemia, diarrhea with bloody feces, and a slow progressive wasting disease.

Because some larvae become encysted in the mother and are activated during pregnancy, newborn puppies and kittens can become infected when they start nursing. In these cases, the mother could test negative for hookworm eggs in the feces because the activated larvae travel to the mammary glands, not through the lungs and into the intestines. The damage caused by adult hookworms will begin early in the life of a newborn host.

HOOKWORMS IN HUMANS

When the infective larvae of hookworms (especially *A. braziliense*) penetrate through minute breaks in the skin of humans, they are unable to complete their migration to the lungs and are trapped in the epidermis layer of skin. They migrate around under the skin in a random fashion. This migration of larvae causes CLM or *creeping eruption* (Figure 20).

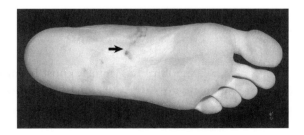

FIGURE 20. Cutaneous larva migrans (creeping eruption) in the sole of a man's foot. (From Hendrix CM, Robinson E: *Diagnostic parasitology for veterinary technicians*, ed 3, St Louis, 2006, Mosby.)

The migration starts at the point of entry, which is frequently in the area between the toes. Symptoms usually appear within 2 weeks of being exposed to the larvae. Patients have often just returned from a tropical area where they were exposed to the larvae. The larval migration appears as a serpentine or linear, single, inflamed, track line. The larvae can travel quickly, often 1 to 2 centimeters per day. Sometimes the larvae will disappear and reappear in another location. Itching may occur, and the patient might also experience pain, local swelling, and sometimes fever. Vesicles containing serous fluid often appear along the tracks. Secondary bacterial infection is common. Eventually the larvae will die, and the condition becomes self-limiting.

CLM is seen most often in children, utility workers who must enter crawl spaces, gardeners, travelers to tropical regions, sunbathers who may become infected in areas other than between the toes, and others exposed to soil or sand contaminated with cat and dog feces.

Diagnosis

DOGS AND CATS
Hookworms are diagnosed by microscopic examination of feces that contain hookworm eggs.

HUMANS
CLM is diagnosed based on lesions and the patient's history.

Treatment

Dogs and cats are treated with antiparasitic drugs to rid them of hookworms.

CLM is often successfully treated with a single dose of an antiparasitic drug. Antibacterial ointments can be used to control the secondary bacterial infection that may develop.

Prevention and Control

Prevention and control of hookworms in pets is based on eliminating the hookworms and controlling access to areas contaminated with hookworm eggs and larvae.

For pets, this involves the following steps:
• Deworm pets on a regular basis. Most veterinary clinics have a protocol that includes treatment or prevention of hookworm infection.

- Puppies and kittens should be examined for hookworms and treated, if necessary, when they are very young. Again, most veterinary clinics will have a protocol for this, usually associated with the vaccination schedule.
- Keep areas where pets defecate clean. Feces should be removed at least once a week and disposed of where animals and people cannot come in contact with them. Feces can be buried or bagged and disposed of with the regular garbage. Freezing will kill the larvae, as will hot, dry conditions.
- Kennels can be cleaned with a solution of 3 cups of household bleach to a gallon of cool water. Remove all fecal material and either spray or mop the solution on the kennel floor.
- Limit the amount of contact your pet has with other animals or animal feces. Keep pets on a leash. With the advent of dog parks, this is becoming more difficult, especially if pet owners do not pick up after their dogs.

Prevention of CLM is based on good hygiene and common sense:

- Do not let children play where dogs and cats may have defecated. Do not let children go barefoot in these areas.
- Wash hands after playing and before eating.
- Do not allow cats to use sandboxes, flower beds, or gardens as litter boxes. Keep the sandboxes covered when not in use.
- Put something between you and the sand when sunbathing. Wear footwear when walking on the beach.
- Keep dogs and cats off beaches as much as possible.
- Clean up dog feces on a regular basis.
- Keep dogs and cats on a regular, preventive worming schedule.

INFLUENZA

Influenza viruses are usually quite host specific, and as such, are not considered zoonotic. Human influenza is a respiratory disease spread among people by aerosol droplets containing the influenza virus or by contact with surfaces contaminated with the virus. Wild migratory birds carry the virus but do not seem to become ill. Avian influenza is spread among domesticated birds, such as chickens, ducks, and turkeys that come in contact with secretions and excretions from infected migratory birds. From time to time, the avian influenza virus will mutate into a virus that can infect people and be spread from person to person easily. This is how pandemic influenza outbreaks are started.

MORBIDITY: +
MORTALITY: + TO +++
ETIOLOGY: VIRAL

All viruses have only one purpose: to replicate. To do this they must invade a host cell and take over the genetic machinery. This allows the virus to replicate until the cell becomes filled with the virus. The newly created viruses then escape from the host cell, destroying the cell in the process, and find their way to other host cells to repeat the process. While in a host cell the virus may undergo minor mutations that make it look different. The mutation results in a new antigenic strain that the host's immune system cannot recognize, even if it was able to recognize the original virus. This is called *antigen drift* and is the reason new flu vaccines have to be created annually. The mutations do not inhibit the virus's pathogenicity. Each strain must have a specific vaccine produced to protect people from infection.

More than one virus can infect the same host cell. When this happens entirely new viruses may appear that have components of each original virus. For example, if an avian influenza virus and a human influenza virus co-infect the same host cell, portions of the two viruses can reassort to create an entirely new virus, not just a new strain. This is called *antigen shift*, and the results are much more serious than those seen with antigen drift. The host species has no previous immunity to this new virus. The dangerous part of this new creation is that it may have the pathogenicity of the avian influenza virus and the ability of the human influenza virus to pass from person to person. This may happen in swine and is how a pandemic could begin (Figure 21).

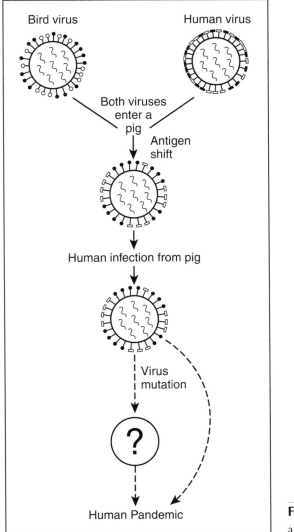

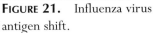

FIGURE 21.   Influenza virus antigen shift.

Influenza viruses are divided into three types: A, B, and C. Type A has been identified in animals and people. Types B and C have been identified in humans only, and are less pathogenic than Type A. Type A presents the greatest zoonotic threat.

The type A influenza virus is divided into subtypes based on the presence of two antigens imbedded on its surface. These antigens create spikes, or protrusions, all over the surface of the virus that allow it to attach to a host cell. The H (hemagglutinin) antigen enables the virus to attach to the host cell, and the N (neuraminidase) antigen allows it to escape from the cell once the virus has replicated many times. Since 16 different H antigens and 9 different N antigens have been identified, there are potentially 144 combinations of H and N antigens. Subtypes are named for the H and N antigens present. For example, the H1N1 influenza virus was responsible for the Spanish Flu pandemic that killed millions of people between 1918 and 1919.

The potential of the H5N1 avian influenza virus to cause a pandemic has been a concern since the mid-1990s. Three conditions must be met before a pandemic can begin:
1. The virus must be in a form for which humans have no inherent immunity.
2. The virus must be pathogenic enough to cause serious illness and death in humans.
3. The virus has to be easily transmitted from person to person.

So far the virus has met the first two conditions. While human cases of H5N1 infection have been relatively low in number and limited to Asia, Africa and Europe, it could be only a matter of time before infections arrive in North America. The mortality rate of H5N1 infection in people is about 70%.

HOSTS

Avian influenza virus subtype A/H5N1 is found mainly in birds.

TRANSMISSION

Transmission of all avian influenza viruses begins with wild birds that carry the virus in their intestines but usually do not get sick from it. Domestic fowl, especially chickens, ducks, and turkeys, are susceptible to infection and may become ill when infected. Transmission to domestic fowl occurs by exposure to secretions and excretions contaminated with the virus, exposure to surfaces contaminated by infected birds, or by direct contact with infected birds.

Rarely, people can become infected by direct contact with an infected bird through handling, slaughtering, defeathering, or preparing the bird for consumption.

H5N1 INFLUENZA IN ANIMALS

So far the H5N1 influenza virus has been confined mainly to birds. The resulting respiratory disease can be so mild as to go unnoticed or so severe that it results in death. It is highly contagious within a flock and can readily be carried from farm to farm by contaminated vehicles, feed, cages, equipment, or clothing.

Pigs are susceptible to both avian and human influenza viruses. If a pig is infected with both an H5N1 avian virus and a highly contagious human influenza virus, the pig could act as a mixing vessel resulting in a new virus through antigen shift. This resulting virus could be an H5N1 strain in pigs that is readily transmitted from person to person, thus providing the third requirement for a pandemic to occur. People may then become infected by handling the infected pigs.

H5N1 INFLUENZA IN HUMANS

The first case of H5N1 influenza infection in humans was reported in Hong Kong in 1997, with 18 confirmed cases and 6 deaths. The clinical signs appear, on average, 7 days after exposure to the virus. Patients will develop lower respiratory tract symptoms, characterized by dyspnea, a hoarse voice, and crackling sounds when they inhale. Most patients will develop pneumonia and multiorgan infection and will deteriorate rapidly. Many patients will die.

DIAGNOSIS

Diagnosis of H5N1 influenza virus infection must be done by virus isolation in a laboratory. The clinical symptoms can resemble the common flu.

TREATMENT

There are four antiviral drugs available, but so far the H5N1 virus has been resistant to two of them. Supportive treatment and treatment of any secondary infections are necessary.

PREVENTION

There is no vaccine available for protection against H5N1, because a strain that will easily spread from person to person has not yet developed. Because we can't predict the make-up of the potential pandemic H5N1 strain, production of a vaccine cannot begin until this strain has been created and the pandemic has begun.

LA CROSSE ENCEPHALITIS

La Crosse encephalitis is a mosquito-borne, viral disease with the potential of infecting the central nervous system in humans, usually children under 15. The disease is named for La Crosse, Wisconsin, where it was first identified in 1963.

MORBIDITY: +
MORTALITY: +
ETIOLOGY: VIRAL

La Crosse encephalitis virus (LCEV) is an arbovirus that causes La Crosse encephalitis (LCE). Other important encephalitis arboviruses include the eastern equine encephalitis virus, St. Louis encephalitis virus, West Nile virus, and western equine encephalitis virus.

HOSTS

Woodland mammals, especially chipmunks and tree squirrels, are the natural hosts for LCEV.

TRANSMISSION

LCE is seen primarily in upper Midwestern, mid-Atlantic, and Southeastern states. LCEV is passed from one woodland mammal to another by the bite of a treehole mosquito. This mosquito breeds in treeholes (the area between the two main trunks of trees with two or more trunks) when rainwater collects there. It also breeds in man-made containers such as old tires, buckets, toys, cans, or anything that can hold water. The treehole mosquito is also found in deciduous forests or shaded areas; they do not fly more than 200 yards from where they were born. Unlike most other mosquitoes, treehole mosquitoes bite during the day.

When a mosquito ingests blood from an infected mammal, the virus replicates in the mosquito and moves to other locations in the mosquito's body, including the salivary glands. When the mosquito takes its next meal on an uninfected mammal, it deposits a small drop of saliva at the bite, which acts as an anticoagulant. The saliva contains the virus, which enters the mammal, replicates, and becomes a source of virus for other mosquitoes that come for a meal. Once infected, the mosquito is infected for life (Figure 22).

Once a mammal is infected, the virus replicates and a viremia develops, making the virus available to mosquitoes. Chipmunks and squirrels are considered amplifiers of LCEV, because one animal can potentially infect many mosquitoes.

Treehole mosquitoes can pass the virus transovarially to the next generation of mosquitoes. Mosquito eggs are laid in treeholes or other man-made containers, just above the water line. The eggs do not hatch until enough water has accumulated to cover the eggs with water. This can happen several times a year or may not happen until the next year. The virus winters over in the eggs.

LCE is transmitted to people by a mosquito that has previously bitten an infected woodland mammal. People are dead-end hosts. Person-to-person transmission does not occur.

LA CROSSE ENCEPHALITIS IN ANIMALS

Woodland mammals and mosquitoes infected with LCEV do not develop any clinical signs of disease. No animals other than humans seem to be affected by LCEV.

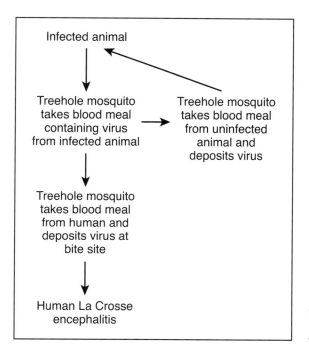

FIGURE 22.   La Crosse encephalitis.

LA CROSSE ENCEPHALITIS IN HUMANS

Many people, especially adults, who become infected with LCEV do not develop clinical signs of illness. In mild encephalitis cases, people may have a fever, headache, nausea, vomiting, mental confusion, and lethargy. This form of LCE is self-limiting within a few days.

In more severe cases, usually seen in children, the virus can enter the central nervous system resulting in more severe signs of encephalitis. This can produce sudden seizures, paralysis, mental confusion, muscle tremors, coma, and brain damage that may be long lasting.

LCE is seen midsummer through early fall. The incubation period is 5 to 15 days. People most at risk for developing LCE are children, people who live in or visit wooded areas, and people who work in wooded areas. People who have containers of standing water on their property may also be at increased risk. The mortality rate is 1 to 3%, and fatalities are seen most often in children.

DIAGNOSIS

Diagnosis is based on the presence of antibodies against LCEV in serum.

TREATMENT

There is no specific drug to combat LCE. Supportive care and management of neurological symptoms are the only medical care available.

PREVENTION

There is no vaccine available for protection against LCE in humans. Prevention centers on decreased exposure to treehole mosquitoes.

Reducing exposure to mosquitoes involves the following steps:
- Drain standing water in old tires, cans, buckets, and other containers, especially after rainfall or watering. These are favorite breeding sites for treehole mosquitoes.
- Reduce forest activities during daytime hours, which are peak hours for treehole mosquito activity.
- Wear protective clothing when going into forests during daytime hours, when the mosquitoes are biting. Protective clothing includes long-sleeved shirts and long pants.
- Use insect repellent containing DEET on exposed skin.

LEPTOSPIROSIS

Leptospirosis is considered one of the most common zoonotic diseases in the world. In humans, it is also known as *Weil's disease*, *swineherd's disease*, *rice-field disease*, *swamp fever*, and *mud fever*. In horses, it can cause a condition known as *periodic ophthalmia*, or *moon blindness*. In dogs it is known as *canicola disease*.

MORBIDITY: +

MORTALITY: +

ETIOLOGY: BACTERIAL

Leptospirosis is caused by bacteria that belong to the genus *Leptospira*. All *Leptospira* are spirochetes (slender, spiral, motile bacteria) that coil around a central axis. They are aerobic gram-negative organisms. They are motile because they are flexible and able to bend and wriggle. They prefer to live in an alkaline environment.

There are two species of *Leptospira* recognized today: *L. interrogans* and *L. biflexa*. *L. interrogans* is pathogenic to humans and animals. *L. biflexa* is nonpathogenic and is free-living in water. *L. interrogans* has over 200 different strains, or *serovars* (species variants), some of which are host-species specific and others that can infect a variety of host species. All of the serovars look identical. Each serovar has a particular host species it prefers, but some of the serovars will infect other species, too. For example, *L. interrogans* serovar *canicola* is found primarily in dogs but will also infect cattle.

HOSTS

Over 160 mammalian species, including humans, have been identified as susceptible to leptospirosis.

TRANSMISSION

Leptospira organisms are passed in the urine of an infected host and are transmitted to another host through mucous membranes and skin lesions. Transmission may occur through exposure to water, soil, or food that has been contaminated with infected urine. The most common mode of transmission is by drinking contaminated water. Catching and eating infected rodents and eating grass and food contaminated with urine are other common modes of transmission among animals. Animals and humans can become infected by touching placentas, aborted fetuses, and related tissues (Figure 23).

When the organism enters the host's body, it enters the blood stream and is distributed throughout the body. Organisms are found in all tissues initially, but eventually primarily in the kidney, liver, spleen, respiratory tract, central nervous system, eyes, and genital tract, where they live and reproduce. Wherever the organism is found, it causes blood vessel damage, primarily in capillaries. Eventually, the organism will be removed from most organs by the host's immune system, but some organisms may remain in the kidneys, eyes, central nervous system, and genital tract and continue reproducing. As in other organs, the capillaries in the kidney are damaged, so blood leaks into the urine and the host passes bloody urine. The liver is the second most commonly affected organ. Liver damage is characterized by jaundice (yellowing of skin and mucous membranes).

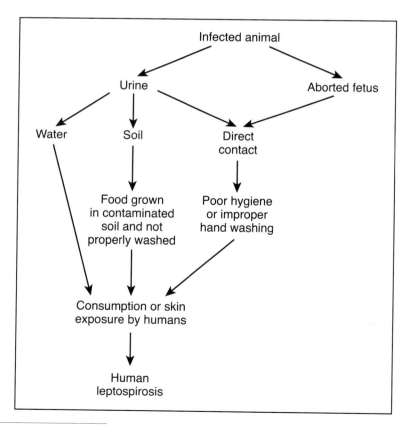

FIGURE 23. Leptospirosis.

LEPTOSPIROSIS IN ANIMALS

Many cases of leptospirosis in animals are subclinical. Some animals, like rodents, carry *Leptospira* organisms and do not become ill but become carrier animals. Some animals that survive leptospirosis will also become carriers. Some host species develop *host-adapted serovars*, which means they will not become sick when infected with a specific serovar.

In all animals, the state of the immune system and age play important roles in determining which animals will become infected. Young animals at or near weaning time are the most susceptible. In pregnant animals the *Leptospira* organisms may cross the placenta and cause abortion, still births, or weakened babies. The severity of leptospirosis in animals depends on which serovar is involved. Animals can become infected with more than one *Leptospira* serovar, each of which will produce different degrees of disease.

DOGS

Initially, dogs with leptospirosis will exhibit several days of fever, abdominal pain, vomiting, depression, muscle pain, anorexia, bloody urine, and diarrhea. These are nonspecific signs, but as the disease progresses, kidney failure and dehydration will develop. Liver damage is indicated by jaundice and bilirubin in the urine. Dogs may stand or walk with a hunched back because of kidney pain.

CATS

Cats rarely show symptoms of leptospirosis, even though many of them have antibodies to the *Leptospira* organism that would indicate prior disease or vaccination.

CATTLE

Some serovars produce few clinical signs in cattle; others are very pathogenic. When there is a pathogenic serovar present, there are two forms of leptospirosis that can manifest in cattle: *acute* and *chronic*.

The acute form strikes young calves and is characterized by anorexia, fever, hemoglobinuria, anemia, and pulmonary congestion, leading to difficult breathing.

The chronic form strikes older cattle and is characterized by abortion, still births, or births of premature, weak calves. Abortions are most common during the third trimester of pregnancy. In dairy cows, there is usually a sudden drop in milk production in infected animals. The milk becomes thick and yellow, with blood tinges.

SHEEP

Leptospirosis in sheep in similar to that in cattle, only less severe.

PIGS

Leptospirosis in pigs is characterized by late-term abortions, occurring some-time during the last month of pregnancy. Piglets that are carried full-term may be born dead or so weak that they die soon after birth. Carrier boars play an important role in transmitting *Leptospira* organisms to sows during mating.

HORSES

Leptospirosis in horses can cause abortion and still births. Kidney failure is rare. Some horses will develop a recurrent uveitis (inflammation in the middle layer of the eye), also known as *periodic ophthalmia*, or *moon blindness*. In such cases the eye is painful, is sensitive to light, may water excessively, and is subject to eyelid muscle spasms, called *blepharospasms*, that keep the eye closed.

LEPTOSPIROSIS IN HUMANS

Most leptospirosis outbreaks are associated with exposure to contaminated water. Most cases occur during the warm, moist, late summer and early fall months in rural areas, because the organisms survive in fresh-water rivers, lakes, and streams; damp, alkaline soil found around river banks; and mud.

Humans are susceptible to all serovars that infect animals but are considered dead-end hosts. The incubation period is somewhere between 2 days and 4 weeks following exposure to a contaminated source. People at risk for infection are those who work with animals, such as veterinarians and veterinary technicians; people who work outdoors or in areas where animals frequently urinate, such as workers on farms and in kennels and pet shops, sewer workers, professionals who work in crawl spaces, and people in the fishing industry; and people who are in and around contaminated water, such as travelers to developing countries or tropical areas, hikers, campers, backpackers, and people who engage in water sports.

The initial signs of leptospirosis resemble the flu and are characterized by fever, chills, vomiting, diarrhea, headache, and muscle aches. The patient may appear to recover and then become sick again. With treatment the disease will last for a few days to 3 weeks. Without treatment it may take months to recover. Because the signs are not specific for leptospirosis, cases are often wrongly diagnosed and underreported. The liver and kidney are not visibly affected in this mild form, and no jaundice is visible. If women are infected during the early months of pregnancy, there is a high rate of spontaneous abortion.

In about 10% of cases, the patient may become seriously ill, with the signs listed above, as well as liver failure, kidney failure, or meningitis. Jaundice is apparent with this form of leptospirosis but not with the milder form. The symptoms come on suddenly and are severe. Other tissues that might be involved include skeletal muscle, the respiratory system, the heart, and the eyes. This more severe form of leptospirosis is known as *Weil's disease*. Weil's disease is a more serious problem in the elderly; the mortality rate can be up to 10%.

DIAGNOSIS

A tentative diagnosis can be made with the patient history and serological testing. A definitive diagnosis is made by growing the organism on culture media. This is sometimes difficult, because the organism has strict growing conditions and grows slowly.

TREATMENT

Leptospirosis is treated with antibiotics. The earlier the treatment is started, the more successful it will be. Periodic ophthalmia in horses is treated topically and systemically. Supportive treatment for other signs, such as dehydration, pain, vomiting, and diarrhea, is also employed.

PREVENTION

There is no vaccine to protect humans or horses against leptospirosis. There are multivalent vaccines available to protect cattle, pigs, and dogs. A multivalent vaccine protects against more than one serovar but not all of them. An animal is still susceptible to infection by a serovar not included in the vaccine.

LISTERIOSIS

Until the 1980s listeriosis was rarely reported in humans but was fairly common in animals. Since then, there have been increased reports of listeriosis in people. In animals listeriosis is also known as *circling disease* or *silage disease*.

MORBIDITY: +
MORTALITY: ++
ETIOLOGY: BACTERIAL

Listeriosis is caused by *Listeria monocytogenes*, a gram-positive, motile, very resistant *coccobacillus*, or oval-shaped rod. It can grow in a wide range of temperatures, from 39° to 111° F. Because it tolerates cooler temperatures, listeriosis is seen more often in temperate and cooler climates. The normal reservoirs of *L. monocytogenes* are soil and the gastrointestinal tracts of mammals. The organism can be killed by pasteurization or cooking, but it can grow in food stored in a refrigerator, in food with a high salt content, and in an acid environment.

HOSTS

L. monocytogenes has been found in mammals, birds, fish, insects, crustaceans, water, milk, cheese, deli meats, hot dogs, sewage, silage, feces, genital secretions, nasal discharges, and soil. In humans, groups that are most affected are pregnant women, newborns, people with compromised immune systems, elderly people, and those taking steroids. These groups are considered high-risk groups. In animals, adult ruminants seem to be most commonly affected. Healthy people and animals rarely get sick if infected with *L. monocytogenes* but can pass the organism in their feces.

TRANSMISSION

L. monocytogenes is spread from animal to animal via the fecal-oral route. An infected animal passes *L. monocytogenes* in its feces, which contaminates vegetation. A susceptible host eats the vegetation and becomes infected. Animals also get infected by eating contaminated silage and hay or by drinking contaminated water. People usually become infected with *L. monocytogenes* by eating food or drinking water that has been contaminated with feces that contain the organism. Some ready-to-eat foods become infected after they have been heat processed (Figure 24).

LISTERIOSIS IN ANIMALS

The most frequently seen form of listeriosis in animals is encephalitis, seen in adult ruminants and, rarely, in adult pigs. Sheep and goats are most susceptible to *L. monocytogenes* infection. The disease is one of winter and spring, because this is a time when animals are confined and fed silage or hay. If either the silage or hay has been contaminated with *L. monocytogenes*, it could be a source of infection to the animals.

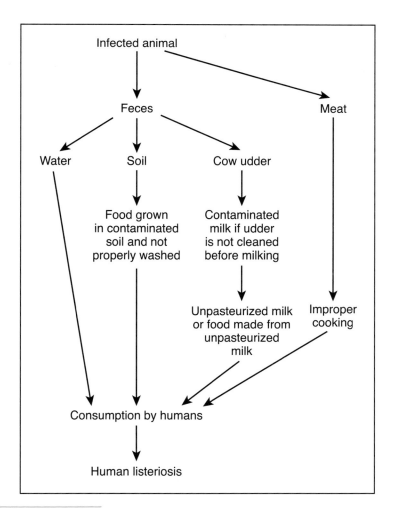

FIGURE 24.   Listeriosis.

The organism enters the body through abrasions in the mouth and travels to the brain, where it causes unilateral encephalitis. The incubation period is about 10 days. The signs exhibited by an infected animal include depression, fever, and incoordination. Infected animals will segregate themselves into corners and frequently are seen leaning against a fence or building. An infected animal may start circling in one direction. The direction is determined by the side of the brain affected (Figure 25). If the facial nerve is affected, it will be unilateral and will be seen as a drooping ear, drooping eyelid, dilated nostril, drooping lower lip, tongue protrusion, excessive salivation, and difficulty eating. As the disease progresses, the animal becomes progressively paralyzed, will fall down on its side and paddle its legs as if running, enter into a coma, and eventually die. The mortality rate can be as high as 70% in sheep. Cattle seem to be a bit more tolerant, but the mortality rate can still reach 50%.

Three other, less common forms of listeriosis in animals are septicemia in monogastric animals and young ruminants, abortion or stillbirths in all animals, and mastitis in ruminants.

The septicemia in monogastric animals has been seen in pigs, dogs, cats, rabbits, and young ruminants, before the rumen is functional. The clinical signs include fever, depression, anorexia, respiratory signs, and diarrhea leading to death. These animals are infected by ingesting or inhaling the organism.

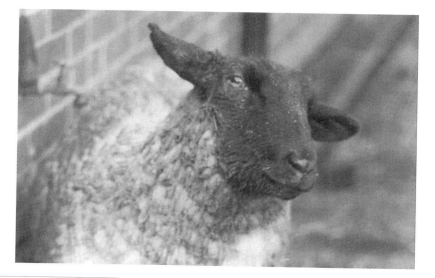

FIGURE 25.   Listeriosis in a sheep showing unilateral facial paralysis. (From Quinn PJ et al: *Clinical veterinary microbiology,* London, 1994, Mosby.)

After the organism gets to the intestines, it migrates through the wall and enters the blood stream, where it is distributed throughout the body. The liver is the principal organ involved.

L. monocytogenes can infect any pregnant animal. It causes fetal deaths, abortions, stillbirths, and death of newborns. Most abortions occur in the last trimester of pregnancy and happen without warning. In this form of listeriosis, the animals are infected by ingesting or inhaling *L. monocytogenes*. After ingestion the organism travels to the uterus, crosses the placenta, and infects the fetus. The organism can be shed in milk and vaginal secretions for up to 2 months following the abortion.

In cattle, mastitis is rarely seen with *L. monocytogenes* infection. When it does occur, it is seen in one quarter only and is not responsive to antibiotic treatment.

LISTERIOSIS IN HUMANS

Healthy adults and children rarely become clinically ill with *L. monocytogenes* infection, though the organism can be found in the feces of healthy individuals. Pregnant women, newborns, elderly people, and people with compromised immune systems are most susceptible to *L. monocytogenes* infection. *L. monocytogenes* most often affects the pregnant uterus, central nervous system, and blood.

People become infected by eating food or drinking water that has been contaminated with *L. monocytogenes*. The foods most commonly incriminated are raw vegetables grown in soil that has been fertilized with contaminated manure; unpasteurized milk or products made from raw milk; uncooked meats; and foods contaminated after processing, such as soft cheese, deli meats, and hotdogs.

The average incubation period is 3 weeks. The clinical signs of listeriosis in humans include initial flulike symptoms of fever, sore muscles, nausea, and diarrhea. If the organism spreads to the central nervous system, these symptoms can be followed by headache, stiff neck, confusion, incoordination, and convulsions. Abscesses can form in the brain. In adults the clinical signs will depend on which organs are affected. Meningitis, pneumonia, abscesses, skin lesions, heart disease, and conjunctivitis have been reported.

The organism can also cross the placenta and infect the fetus, resulting in abortion if the infection occurs in early pregnancy, or stillbirths and babies who are born with listeriosis if the infection occurs later in pregnancy. Babies who are infected near term or at birth do not eat, are lethargic, become jaundiced and may vomit and develop skin lesions and meningitis. They have a nearly 50% mortality rate. Some babies do not show signs for about a week. In these later-developing cases, meningitis is the most common manifestation of listeriosis. If babies survive the infection, they may have long-term neurological problems and may not develop normally.

DIAGNOSIS

The only way to definitively diagnose listeriosis is to culture and identify *L. monocytogenes*. In humans, the tissues cultured include blood, cerebral spinal fluid, and feces. In aborted fetuses, the placenta, feces, and gastrointestinal contents may be cultured. In animals, the preferred samples are brain tissue or aborted fetuses and associated tissues. Suspect food can also be cultured. *L. monocytogenes* is difficult to grow and requires special culture media. Faster methods of diagnosis are being investigated.

TREATMENT

Listeriosis is treated with antibiotics. The earlier the treatment is started, the more effective it will be, but even if treatment has been started, death can occur. In people, this is especially true in the elderly, fetuses and newborns, and people with compromised immune systems. Supportive treatment is also administered and is determined by the signs and symptoms being exhibited.

PREVENTION

Vaccines for listeriosis are not available in the United States. Prevention recommendations for listeriosis in humans are generally the same as for any food-borne disease. These recommendations include:
- Cook all meat thoroughly.
- Thoroughly wash foods that will be eaten raw.
- Separate raw meats from other food.
- Do not drink unpasteurized milk or eat food made from unpasteurized milk.
- Wash cutting boards, knives, utensils, and hands after handling raw meat or other uncooked foods.
- High-risk individuals should not eat hotdogs, deli meat, or luncheon meats unless they have been heated until steaming hot; salads at a salad bar and foods with a high water content should also be avoided.
- High-risk individuals should not eat soft cheeses, unless such cheeses are specifically labeled as made from pasteurized milk.
- High-risk individuals should not eat refrigerated meat spreads, because *L. monocytogenes* can grow at refrigerator temperatures.

- High-risk people should not eat refrigerated smoked meats, often labeled as *lox*, *smoked*, *jerky*, *kippered*, or *nova-style*.
- People who are working around aborted fetuses, or those who perform animal autopsies, called *necropsies*, should handle tissue carefully. Pregnant women should avoid handling such tissues altogether.

In animals, the best prevention is to minimize the chance of infection. Sick animals should be isolated as soon as clinical signs appear. Dead animals should be removed from the premises immediately. All buildings where affected animals have lived should be cleaned and disinfected, and any bedding should be burned. Check silage for spoilage, and discontinue feeding contaminated silage.

LYME DISEASE

Lyme disease is a bacterial infection that affects many systems in the body. It is transmitted by tick bites and has become the most common arthropod-borne, human disease in the United States.

MORBIDITY: +
MORTALITY: +
ETIOLOGY: BACTERIAL

Borrelia burgdorferi is the bacterium responsible for Lyme disease. It is a spirochete, which means it is a spiral-shaped bacterium that is longer than it is wide. *B. burgdorferi* has very specific growth requirements in the laboratory, so it is not routinely cultured.

HOSTS

The two primary reservoir hosts for *B. burgdorferi* are white-footed mice and whitetail deer. Even though the ticks bite the deer, the deer do not become infected, but they serve as means of survival and transportation for the ticks. Humans and other animals, such as dogs, cats, horses, and cattle, can also become infected with *B. burgdorferi*.

TRANSMISSION

Ticks transmit *B. burgdorferi* through their bites, from one host to another. The organism lives in the intestinal tract of the tick and can be passed from host to host when the tick feeds. It takes 24 to 36 hours after a tick becomes attached to its host before it starts releasing *B. burgdorferi*.

The tick life cycle has three active stages after the egg hatches: larva, nymph, and adult (see Appendix 1). The larva must have a blood meal before it can molt to the nymph stage, and the nymph must have a blood meal before it can molt to the adult stage. A tick at each active stage can become infected when it takes a blood meal. The bacteria stay with the tick when it molts to the next stage. As it feeds before molting, a tick at each stage can infect another animal by depositing *B. burgdorferi* at the site of its bite. Typically the larva will feed on small rodents, like the white-footed mouse. If the mouse was infected, the larva becomes infected. Nymphs prefer feeding on many animals, such as small rodents, dogs, cats, horses, cattle, and humans. Similarly, if any of these animals were infected, the nymph would become infected. Adult ticks prefer to feed on whitetail deer. The life cycle takes 2 years to complete. Ticks can feed on people at any of the three stages (Figure 26).

Two ticks that can transmit Lyme disease to humans have been identified: the black-legged deer tick, *Ixodes scapularis*, in the northeastern and north central United States, and the western black-legged tick, *Ixodes pacificus*, on the Pacific coast of the United States. The larvae of both black-legged ticks are the size of a pin head and are tan colored. The nymphs are the size of a poppy seed and are beige or semitransparent. The adults are about the size of an apple

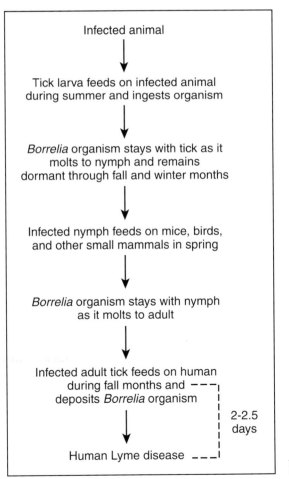

FIGURE 26.   Lyme disease.

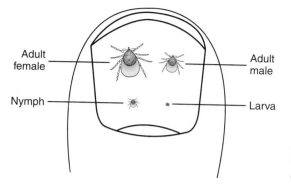

Adult female

Adult male

Nymph

Larva

FIGURE 27.   Adult female deer tick on a finger.

seed and are black or reddish (Figure 27). For Lyme disease to occur, there must be *B. burgdorferi*, white-footed mice, and whitetail deer in an area.

Dogs and cats can get Lyme disease but cannot transfer it directly to people. They can, however, transport ticks into a home, yard, kennel, or veterinary facility.

Not all black-legged ticks are infected with *B. burgdorferi*. In some areas less than 1% of the ticks are infected, but in other areas over 50% are. *B. burgdorferi* can infect other species of ticks, but none of them have been shown to transmit Lyme disease to humans.

LYME DISEASE IN ANIMALS

Many animals infected with *B. burgdorferi* do not develop clinical signs. If they do develop an illness, it may be a long time after the initial infection.

CATS
Cats that develop Lyme disease usually display fever, anorexia, lethargy, lameness, and irregular breathing. There is nothing about these symptoms that is specific to Lyme disease, so many cases will go undiagnosed.

DOGS
Dogs develop a lameness that shifts from one leg to another, fever, anorexia, kidney damage, heart problems, and possibly central nervous system involvement expressed as aggression, seizures, or mental confusion. Transplacental transmission has been documented.

CATTLE
Cattle frequently do not exhibit any signs of Lyme disease when they become infected. They may develop lameness, laminitis, fever, and swollen joints. A rash may develop on the udder. *B. burgdorferi* has been found in colostrum,

blood, milk, synovial fluid, and aborted fetal tissue in cows. Freezing does not kill the organism, but pasteurization does.

HORSES
Horses will develop lameness, laminitis, painful or stiff joints, and anorexia. They seldom develop a fever with Lyme disease. Spontaneous abortion and encephalitis are sometimes reported. The central nervous system may become involved, resulting in difficulty swallowing, head tilt, or aimless wandering. Transplacental transmission has been reported.

LYME DISEASE IN HUMANS

Most cases of Lyme disease in people occur during the spring and summer months. The disease follows a predictable progression. If not diagnosed and treated early in its course, it becomes a three-stage disease.

Stage one is the *early, localized stage*. It usually starts with flulike symptoms, followed by a rash developing 3 days to 1 month after infection. The rash, known as *erythema migrans* (EM), starts at the site of a tick bite. It can be a solid, red rash that expands, or it can take on a *bull's-eye* or *target* appearance, appearing as a central red spot, surrounded by normal skin that is surrounded by an expanding red rash (Figure 28). The rash can remain small, or it can spread to an area the size

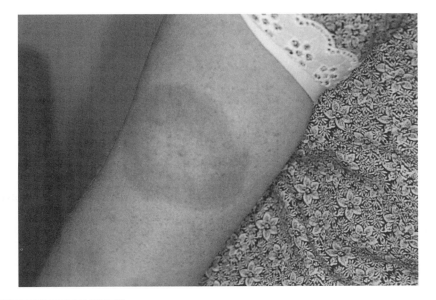

FIGURE 28.   Typical "bull's-eye" or "target" rash seen with Lyme disease in humans. (From Murray PR et al: *Medical microbiology*, ed 4, St Louis, 2002, Mosby.)

of a person's back. In dark-skinned people, the rash resembles a bruise. The *B. burgdorferi* spirochetes can be isolated from the leading edge of the rash. This distinctive rash is unique to Lyme disease, but does not develop in some cases. The rash should not be confused with the allergic reaction that sometimes develops from tick saliva at the site of a tick bite. The allergic reaction occurs within a few hours, does not spread, and will disappear in a few days.

Stage two is the *early, disseminated stage*. During this stage, which begins 2 weeks to 3 months after infection, the bacteria enter the bloodstream and are spread to various sites in the body. Symptoms that may be seen during this stage are fever, sore throat, fatigue, enlarged lymph nodes, tingling or numbness in the extremities, stiff neck, headache, migrating joint pain, mild nervous system involvement, and rashes beyond the site of the bite. Facial paralysis that resembles Bell's palsy, a condition that causes the facial muscles to weaken or become paralyzed due to cranial nerve trauma, may develop.

Stage three is the *persistent infection stage*. If Lyme disease is not diagnosed in the earlier stages, stage three will occur any time from weeks to years after infection. Symptoms include arthritis, especially in the knees, which manifests as brief episodes of pain and swelling, and nervous system involvement which may include numbness, meningitis, or severe headache. Irregular heart rhythms may develop.

DIAGNOSIS

Diagnosis is based on the distinctive rash that appears up to a month after a tick bite. If the rash does not develop, diagnosis must be based on the history and evidence of a tick bite. In some cases in which the rash does not develop, the first sign of Lyme disease may be arthritis or nervous system disorders.

Serological tests are not valid until 1 month after infection.

TREATMENT

Antibiotics are used to treat Lyme disease. Starting the treatment early will result in higher success rates. In the early stage, oral antibiotics are administered for 3 to 4 weeks, and recovery is usually complete and uneventful. If diagnosis is not made until later in the disease process, the treatment may have to include intravenous antibiotics, will probably have to last longer, and will probably have a lower success rate.

PREVENTION

There is a vaccine available for dogs but not for humans.

Tick control products, such as tick collars, should be used on pets that can possibly be exposed to ticks.

The best prevention is to decrease exposure to ticks by following these guidelines (see Appendix 2):

- Avoid areas where ticks thrive as much as possible. May, June, and July are months when ticks are still immature and harder to see because of their light color. These are also the months when people are most active outdoors.
- Ticks have to live where their hosts live, so areas where white-footed mice and whitetail deer live are where ticks are found. These places can include lawns, gardens, wooded areas, overgrown brush, tall grass, woodpiles, and leaf litter.
- Wear light-colored clothing when entering an area that may be a habitat for ticks. This will make the adult ticks easier to see and remove before they become attached.
- Wear long-sleeved shirts and long pants tucked into socks so the ticks cannot crawl under clothing; wear high rubber boots and a hat for the same reason.
- Walk in the center of trails to avoid vegetation where ticks are lurking. Ticks cannot fly, jump, skip, or hop, so they must come in direct contact with a host before they can attach themselves. Immature ticks are found hiding in the shade in a moist area. Adult ticks cling to grass, bushes, and shrubs and wait for a host to come by.
- Exposed skin and clothing can be protected with insect repellents containing DEET. Clothes, but not exposed skin, can be protected with insect repellents containing permethrin, which kills ticks on contact.
- Check often for ticks while outside. Black-legged ticks are tiny and easy to miss.
- Do not sit on the ground or on stone walls, where ticks can abound.
- Make daily checks of the entire body for ticks. Look especially in areas where ticks like to attach, such as behind the ears, the back of the neck, in the armpits, behind the knees, and in the groin area. Bathing will remove crawling ticks but will not detach ticks already attached.
- Wash and dry outdoor clothing in hot temperatures after use.
- Remove ticks as soon as they are found. It takes 24 to 36 hours after a tick becomes attached before it starts releasing *B. burgdorferi*.
- To remove a tick, use fine tweezers, grasp the tick as close to the skin as possible, and pull straight back with a slow, steady force. Avoid crushing the tick's body. Kill the tick by dropping it in alcohol. Save the tick in alcohol as a possible diagnostic aid.

LYMPHOCYTIC CHORIOMENINGITIS

Lymphocytic choriomeningitis (LCM) is a viral disease spread from rodents to other rodents and humans. LCM can have serious effects on human fetuses during the first two trimesters and on people with suppressed immune systems.

MORBIDITY: +

MORTALITY: +

ETIOLOGY: VIRAL

LCM is caused by the lymphocytic choriomeningitis virus (LCMV).

HOSTS

The natural host for LCMV is the wild house mouse. Other rodents become infected by exposure to the house mouse. Pet mice, hamsters, and guinea pigs have also been identified as sources of infection for people. Less commonly infected animals are chinchillas, rats, rabbits, dogs, pigs, and primates.

TRANSMISSION

LCMV is found in the feces, urine, saliva, semen, milk, and blood of infected rodents. It is also found in their nesting or bedding materials. Rodents and people become infected by coming in contact with any of these excretions. Transmission can occur through inhalation of aerosolized virus on dried material, by consumption, or through direct contact with the excretions. No person-to-person transmission has been documented, except for vertical transmission from mother to fetus. There has been one case reported of four people developing LCM after receiving organ transplants from a single donor who had purchased a pet hamster just before he died.

LYMPHOCYTIC CHORIOMENINGITIS IN ANIMALS

Most rodents infected with LCMV are lifetime carriers and are not clinically affected by the virus.

LYMPHOCYTIC CHORIOMENINGITIS IN HUMANS

As more people adopt small pets called *pocket pets* (because many of them will fit in a pocket), there are more pet rodents ending up in households.

Many healthy people, nearly one-third of those infected with LCMV, will not develop any symptoms of illness. For healthy people who do become ill, nearly half of them will develop only mild symptoms, with no neurological involvement.

People who become more ill with LCM will develop a two-phase disease. The first phase is called the *initial viremia stage*. Symptoms appear 1 to 2 weeks after exposure to LCMV and include nonspecific, flulike symptoms, such as fever, lethargy, muscle pain, nausea and vomiting, headache, sore throat, and a nonproductive cough. This phase lasts up to a week.

The second phase of LCM is called the *secondary viremia stage*, which develops as the patient seems to recover from the first phase. It is characterized by a more severe headache, a stiff neck, and encephalitis, which is characterized by drowsiness, fever, confusion, nausea, and/or paralysis.

LCM has been associated with a buildup of fluid on the brain, leading to hydrocephalus, which requires surgical release.

Women who become infected with LCMV during the first two trimesters of pregnancy can pass the virus to the fetus. This can result in fetal death or congenital problems such as hydrocephalus, microcephaly, or chorioretinitis.

People with suppressed immune systems, including people with HIV/AIDS, people receiving chemotherapy, organ transplant recipients, and people using steroids are at greater risk for developing a more severe illness.

Some patients have a prolonged recovery, which may last several months. During this time they may experience headaches, fatigue, and dizziness.

DIAGNOSIS

The diagnosis of LCM is based on a patient history of rodent exposure in the previous 1 to 2 weeks and serum immunological testing to identify antibodies against LCMV.

TREATMENT

There is no specific treatment for LCM. Hospitalization may be required, during which supportive therapy, based on the symptoms and the severity of the symptoms, will be administered.

PREVENTION

LCM is best prevented by taking precautions around wild and pet mice:

- Block any access areas wild mice have to the home.
- Set mouse traps for wild mice. Wear gloves when handling dead (or live) mice.
- Protect food from wild mice.
- Do not provide convenient nesting places for wild mice. Keep pet food in secure containers.
- Have wild mice professionally removed if the infestation is great.
- Wipe up mouse droppings by first wetting them down with a dilute bleach solution ($^1/_4$ cup bleach in a gallon of water). Do not sweep or vacuum the droppings, as this may release aerosolized virus particles. Wipe up the wet droppings with disposable towels.
- Clean bedding, cages, dishes, toys, and water bottles used by pet rodents on a regular basis. Wear rubber gloves. If you have more than one cage to clean, disinfect the rubber gloves between each cage.
- If you have more than one cage of pet rodents, do not interchange their cages, toys, food dishes, or water bottles. This could lead to infection spreading from one rodent to another.
- Do not clean cages or other equipment used by pet rodents in the kitchen or any place food is prepared.
- Disinfect any sink or tub used for cleaning cages or equipment with a mild bleach solution when cleaning is completed. Make sure the room is well ventilated.
- Prevent pet mice or other rodents from coming in contact with wild mice or wild mice secretions.
- Diligently wash hands with warm soapy water, or a hand sanitizer if no soap is available, after handling pet rodents or any of their cages, food dishes, etc. Teach children to wash their hands after playing with pet mice, hamsters, and guinea pigs.

MYCOBACTERIUM INFECTIONS (TUBERCULOSIS)

Tuberculosis (TB) is the most common bacterial cause of death in the world. Worldwide, it is the leading cause of death in HIV/AIDS patients. In the United States cases of TB have decreased to an all-time low, but cases are reported every year.

Other names for TB include *consumption* (the disease seemed to consume people from within), *red death* (for the bloody vomiting often seen), *wasting disease*, *white plague* (infected people become very pale), *prosector's wart* (skin TB, transferred by contact with contaminated carcasses), and *Koch's disease* (named for Robert Koch, who discovered the TB organism). Edgar Allen Poe wrote a short story, "The Masque of the Red Death," which deals with TB.

MORBIDITY: +

MORTALITY: +

ETIOLOGY: BACTERIAL

Bacteria belonging to the genus *Mycobacterium* are responsible for TB. The three most important species are *M. bovis* (reservoirs are cattle, dogs, and pigs), *M. avium* (reservoirs are birds, pigs, and sheep), and *M. tuberculosis* (human reservoir). Nonzoonotic *Mycobacterium leprae* causes human leprosy.

Mycobacterium organisms are slow-growing, gram-positive, acid-fast, aerobic bacilli.

HOSTS

Humans are the ultimate reservoir for *M. tuberculosis*, but other animals, such as nonhuman primates, cattle, dogs, pigs, and psittacine birds, can become infected by a process known as *reverse zoonosis*. Cattle will test positive for TB when infected with *M. tuberculosis*, but generally will not become clinically ill. Pigs can become infected by eating table scraps from the table of an infected person. Granulomatous lesions develop in the gastrointestinal tract and associated lymph nodes. Dogs can develop granulomas in any part of the body, but if the pharynx is infected, the organism can be transferred back to people. Birds develop skin granulomas when infected with *M. tuberculosis*. Asian elephants in the United States have tested positive for *M. tuberculosis* and are presumably infected by their handlers. Elephants and handlers have to be tested annually.

M. avium is becoming a concern because of its increased appearance in immunocompromised people, especially HIV/AIDS patients. Birds, pigs and sheep are naturally susceptible to *M. avium* infection. Cattle, dogs, and cats appear to be resistant.

M. bovis is found primarily in cattle and buffalo, but will infect dogs, pigs, and humans.

TRANSMISSION

The *Mycobacterium* species that cause TB are spread by aerosol droplets, contact with infected animals, contact with contaminated surfaces, and ingestion. *M. bovis* can be transmitted to people through unpasteurized milk and products made with unpasteurized milk. Aerosol droplets can be dispersed through talking, singing, laughing, coughing, or sneezing.

TUBERCULOSIS IN ANIMALS

Bovine TB (*M. bovis*) is seen more often in other parts of the world, but despite an eradication program, cases are still being reported in the United States and Canada. In cattle TB can be a chronic, debilitating disease or an acute, rapidly progressing disease. It all depends on the health of the animal's immune system and the dose of bacterium. The early stages of TB are usually asymptomatic, but the later stages are characterized by a low fever, decreased milk production, progressive emaciation, weakness, and anorexia. With respiratory involvement there will be a moist cough that is worse in the morning, during exercise, or during cold weather. Dyspnea and tachypnea may also be evident. Lymph nodes may become swollen, and in some cases, rupture. Enlarged lymph nodes can obstruct blood vessels, the digestive tract, or airways, leading to further complications.

Asymptomatic animals may become symptomatic with old age or stress.

TUBERCULOSIS IN HUMANS

TB was a common disease in people before the advent of pasteurization. Pasteurization kills the TB organisms, so now only sporadic cases are seen in North America. If people are infected via the aerosol droplet mode, signs include a productive cough, fever, cachexia, bloody sputum, and chest pain.

If infection outside the respiratory system (extrapulmonary infection) occurs, clinical signs will reflect the organs involved. The central nervous system and blood vascular system are sometimes affected with extrapulmonary TB. People at risk of developing TB are those who are caring for infected animals, those who perform necropsies on animals that died of TB, HIV/AIDS patients, and those who consume unpasteurized milk or dairy products.

Some people who are exposed to TB organisms do not become ill because their immune systems prevent the bacteria from multiplying. This is known as *latent TB*. The organisms are not eliminated from the body, just put in a state of hibernation. Some time later in life, the organisms may become virulent again and cause active TB. This can happen when the immune system is compromised.

Nonhuman primates can develop TB. They may die suddenly, while appearing to be in good condition, or they may develop classic signs of TB.

DIAGNOSIS

Diagnosis in cattle and people is based on the TB skin test. This is usually performed by injecting a small amount of tuberculin (a sterile liquid containing a nonpathogenic derivative of the *Mycobacterium* bacterium used in the diagnosis of tuberculosis) under the superficial layers of the skin. After 48 to 72 hours, the site is examined. A positive skin test results in a raised bump at the point of injection. The size of this spot determines whether the skin test is considered significant.

A positive reaction indicates the person has been infected with TB. However, there is a difference between being infected with TB organisms and having TB disease. A person may have been exposed to the TB organisms but developed a latent infection. The immune system is preventing the organisms from multiplying, and the person is not clinically ill. While the immune system keeps the organisms in check, these people cannot spread TB. Someone with the clinical disease may be able to spread the disease to other people or animals. A positive skin test must be followed up with further tests (e.g., chest radiographs, sputum tests) in people. Advanced TB or HIV/AIDS may cause the skin test to read falsely negative. Treatment may be necessary.

Cattle that test positive are either isolated or culled from a herd. All other animals that had contact with the infected animal must also be tested.

All cases of bovine TB must be reported to local, state, and federal health departments.

TREATMENT

In most cases treatment using a combination of approved antimicrobials is successful; treatment can last up to 6 months. Untreated cases of TB can be fatal.

PREVENTION

There is a human vaccine available to protect people against TB, but it does not provide 100% protection in adults. If it does provide protection, the protection lasts only about 15 years. The vaccine also can interfere with the skin test.

People at high risk for being exposed to or developing TB can take a drug that will prevent active disease. It is given every day for 6 to 12 months.

Control measures include:

- Educating the public about transmission methods and prevention.
- Not drinking unpasteurized milk or eating products made from unpasteurized milk.
- Wearing protective clothing when handling suspect animals or carcasses.
- Working in a controlled environment when working with *Mycobacterium* organisms in a laboratory setting.
- A regular surveillance program to identify infected people and animals.
- Isolation and quarantine of suspect animals.
- Providing adequate ventilation in areas where TB is known to exist.
- Using ultraviolet light to sanitize the air in hospitals where TB patients are housed. Special respirators and masks must be used by individuals at risk, and TB patients must be isolated in special rooms with controlled ventilation to prevent spread of the organisms.

PASTEURELLOSIS

Animal-bite pasteurellosis is an acute wound infection resulting from exposure to *Pasteurella multocida*. There have been more than 130 disease-causing organisms identified from infected animal bites in people. Pasteurellosis is the most common bite-associated infection.

MORBIDITY: ++
MORTALITY: +
ETIOLOGY: BACTERIAL

Animal-bite pasteurellosis is caused by *P. multocida*, a small, gram-positive coccobacillus. There are other *Pasteurella* species that cause various diseases in animals, but *P. multocida* is the most common zoonotic species.

HOSTS

P. multocida is part of the normal flora in the respiratory and digestive tracts of many warm-blooded animals. The presence of *P. multocida* in these animals usually does not cause illness. Cats and dogs are the most common source of animal-bite pasteurellosis. Some rats also carry *P. multocida* in their mouths, which can cause wound infection.

TRANSMISSION

P. multocida is usually transferred from the mouth of a cat or dog through a bite wound or contact of the animal's saliva with broken skin (e.g., scratch, abrasion, cut). Cat bites account for around 90% of infected bites because their sharp teeth puncture the skin more deeply, making the wound harder to clean and creating an environment that favors bacterial growth. Dogs have a more crushing bite that does not result in such a deep bite wound. Animal-bite pasteurellosis has also been caused by contact with saliva from rabbits, cattle, sheep, and rats.

PASTEURELLOSIS IN ANIMALS

Pasteurella spp. are part of the normal flora of the respiratory and digestive tracts of many species of warm-blooded animals. They do not cause illness in healthy animals. When an animal becomes stressed, the nonpathogenic organisms can sometimes become pathogenic, causing primarily respiratory and digestive diseases that are not zoonotic. Cats and dogs can develop wound infections from fighting with other animals.

Pasteurellosis in Humans

Animal-bite pasteurellosis is an acute infection. It is characterized by signs of inflammation around a bite wound or broken skin 2 to 12 hours after exposure if the wound is not properly cleansed. The infected area becomes red, swollen, and painful. There may be a clear or bloody discharge present, and abscesses may develop. Some infected wounds heal slowly.

Most animal bites are found on the hands, arms, neck, face, and legs. Cat bites to the hand are especially dangerous, because the bones, joints, ligaments, and tendons are close to the skin and are more susceptible to puncture injury from a bite. When this happens, serious complications such as septic arthritis or osteomyelitis can occur. Dog bites to the face and neck area can cause bone fractures. This can lead to central nervous system infections.

If animal-bite pasteurellosis develops and is not treated right away, the infection can spread from the area of the bite throughout the body. This can cause serious complications such as abscesses, arthritis, and meningitis.

Anyone can develop animal-bite pasteurellosis if a wound is not properly cleansed. People who are most at risk for developing an infection are young children; the elderly; those with circulatory problems or liver disease; those who have had their spleens removed; or immunocompromised people such as HIV/AIDS patients, organ transplant recipients, people receiving chemotherapy, or those on long-term steroid therapy.

Diagnosis

The initial diagnosis of animal-bite pasteurellosis is based on a history of animal exposure and an acute inflammatory response at the site of exposure, usually a bite wound or a scratch or cut that has been licked by an animal. If the inflammation appears more than 24 hours after exposure, a different organism is probably involved. A definitive diagnosis is based on wound culture to identify *P. multocida*. Samples for culture must be taken before drug therapy is started.

Treatment

Treatment starts with thoroughly cleansing the wound. It is important to scrub the wound several times, over a period of several minutes, using soap under warm, running water. Use a scrub brush if one is available; this will get rid of as much of the bacteria-laden saliva as possible. Follow the scrubbing with an antiseptic solution, such as iodine or Betadine (povidone-iodine solution).

If inflammation develops in spite of a thorough cleansing, an appropriate antibiotic can be administered. The appropriate antibiotic is determined by wound culturing and by an antibiotic sensitivity test of the bacterial isolates by placing antibiotic impregnated disks on the culture medium to determine which antibiotics will inhibit bacterial growth.

A tetanus booster should be given if the patient is not currently protected. If a person was bitten by a wild, stray, or unvaccinated animal, the possibility of rabies must be considered.

PREVENTION

There is no vaccine available to protect against animal-bite pasteurellosis.

To avoid getting bitten, use proper restraint methods when handling animals. In a veterinary clinic or hospital setting, it is unwise to let owners restrain their animals during any procedure. Avoid contact with stray animals, which may be more likely to bite when provoked or handled, and take time to thoroughly cleanse every wound from an animal bite.

PLAGUE

Plague is an acute, highly infectious disease transmitted to humans and animals by the bite of a rat flea. It has been known as *bubonic plague* and *black death*.

MORBIDITY: +
MORTALITY: + TO +++
ETIOLOGY: BACTERIAL

Plague is caused by *Yersinia pestis*, a gram-negative, bipolar-staining rod. *Y. pestis* is easily destroyed by drying or sunlight. It can survive for up to an hour when released into the air. *Y. pestis* is considered a potential biological weapon in aerosol form.

HOSTS

Rats, prairie dogs, rock squirrels, ground squirrels, chipmunks, and other burrowing rodents are the primary reservoirs for *Y. pestis*. Many species of fleas can act as vectors for *Y.* pestis, but the rat flea is the most important vector for the plague bacterium. Ticks and human lice have also been identified as possible vectors. In North America, where the plague is mostly seen in the western third of the United States and Canada, the ground squirrel, rock squirrel, and their fleas are the most common source of human infection. Rats and their fleas have not played a role in plague epidemics in the United States since the Los Angeles epidemic of 1924-1925. Fleas can readily infect cats and, less frequently, dogs. If cats develop a pneumonic plague, they can become a source of infection for people through aerosol transmission of the bacteria on droplets expelled during coughing. Cats, dogs, and rabbits can also bring the infected fleas into a home.

TRANSMISSION

Plague is characterized by periodic outbreaks in a rodent population. A flea transmits *Y. pestis* bacteria from one animal to another or to humans. When a flea takes a blood meal from an infected host, such as a ground squirrel, it also ingests some of the bacteria that are living in the blood of that host. The bacteria stay in the intestines of the flea, and when it takes another meal it deposits some of the *Y. pestis* organisms into a new host (Figure 29).

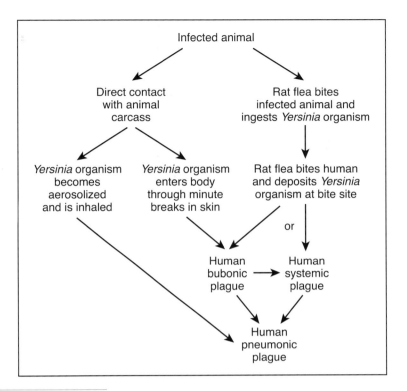

FIGURE 29.   Plague.

In a population of rodents, some of the rodents are resistant to *Y. pestis* infection, and others are highly susceptible. As the susceptible rodents become infected and die, the rodent population decreases, and the fleas will look to other animals, or people, as a blood source.

Transmission can also occur when a person or animal with *pneumonic plague*, which occurs when *Y. pestis* infects the lungs, coughs near another person or animal. The organisms ride on the droplets produced by the cough and are inhaled by another host.

A third method of transmission involves handling infected animals or carcasses. If the animal is infected, some of the bacteria could enter the human body through breaks in the skin. Hunters skinning animals are at risk for this type of transmission.

PLAGUE IN ANIMALS

Some resistant rodents will carry *Y. pestis* and show no symptoms. Other rodents that are more susceptible will develop a fatal disease from

Y. pestis infection. The resistant rodents are the reservoir for the plague bacterium.

Cats will be severely affected by *Y. pestis* infection. They can develop all three forms of plague. The symptoms include fever, abcess formation, lymphadenopathy, hemorrhagic pneumonia, and encephalitis. The disease is fatal in about half of the cats that become infected. Cats can transmit pneumonic plague to people.

Dogs seem to be somewhat resistant to *Y. pestis* infection. If they do become ill, it will be a brief, self-limiting disease. The only symptoms may be fever or lymphadenopathy.

Fleas act as vectors for the plague, and as such, are not affected by the presence of *Y. pestis.*

PLAGUE IN HUMANS

Human outbreaks of plague occur in areas where there is poor housing, usually accompanied by poor sanitation conditions. Other people at risk for coming in contact with the plague bacterium are veterinarians and veterinary technicians; laboratory workers; cat owners; hunters, campers, and hikers; and people who live, work, or play in endemic areas.

Depending on circumstances, three forms of plague may develop separately or in combination.

Bubonic plague is the most common form of plague. It occurs when an infected flea bites a person or when *Y. pestis* enters otherwise, through a break in the skin. The incubation period is 2 to 6 days. Symptoms begin with the sudden onset of headache, chills, and high fever. People may also exhibit body aches, exhaustion, and diarrhea. Small vesicles or abscesses may develop at the site of infection. Swollen, blackened, extremely tender lymph glands, called *buboes*, develop in the area near the bite or skin lesion. The lymph glands contain many *Y. pestis* organisms. The most common areas for buboes to appear are the groin, armpits, or neck. They are usually unilateral. Bubonic plague does not spread from person to person. When left untreated, the mortality rate can approach 75%.

Pneumonic plague occurs when *Y. pestis* infects the lungs. This highly contagious type of plague can spread from person to person through the air, especially in crowded conditions. The incubation period is 1 to 3 days. Transmission can take place if someone breathes in aerosolized bacteria. Pneumonic plague is also spread by breathing in *Y. pestis* suspended in respiratory droplets from a person (or animal) with pneumonic plague.

Becoming infected in this way usually requires direct and close contact with the sick person or animal. The symptoms include acute, overwhelming pneumonia, accompanied by fever and chills; cough; chest pain; dyspnea; and purulent or hemorrhagic sputum. Pneumonic plague may also develop if a person with bubonic or septicemic plague is not treated, allowing the bacteria to spread to the lungs. When left untreated, the mortality rate can be as high as 90%.

Septicemic plague occurs when plague bacteria multiply in the blood. It can be a complication of pneumonic or bubonic plague, or it can occur by itself. When it occurs alone, it is caused in the same ways as bubonic plague; however, buboes do not develop. Patients have fever, chills, prostration, abdominal pain, vomiting, diarrhea, shock, and bleeding into skin and other organs. There is a high mortality rate associated with this type of plague. Septicemic plague does not spread from person to person.

DIAGNOSIS

In people, a tentative diagnosis is based on patient history of a flea bite, exposure to an infected animal, and clinical signs, especially if buboes are present.

Tissue specimens or fluids can be cultured for the presence of *Y. pestis*, and serologic testing can be used to detect antibodies. Because the bacteria can be spread so easily by air, careful precautions must be taken when handling potential *Y. pestis*–infected specimens or fluids.

Any suspected cases of plague must be reported to local, state, and federal health officials. Often the definitive diagnosis comes from the CDC.

TREATMENT

Antibiotics and supportive therapy are the most effective treatment for plague. Treatment must be started within 24 hours of the appearance of the first symptoms to provide the best chance of survival. Patients must be hospitalized and isolated from the general population. Plague can be highly contagious.

PREVENTION

It is virtually impossible to completely control the wild rodent population and equally impossible to control the fleas that feed on them. Prevention is based on controlling rodent populations in rural and urban settings as much as possible and includes:

- Making buildings rodent-proof by plugging any access holes.
- Clearing brush, rock piles, and junk from properties.
- Removing possible rodent food sources, such as pet food left outside.
- Having properties professionally treated to remove fleas.
- Wearing protective clothing and gloves when working with or around any potentially infected animal.
- Keeping dogs and cats away from animal burrows and not allowing pets to eat carcasses of dead rodents or rabbits.
- Using preventive measures to keep fleas off dogs and cats.

Preventive antibiotic therapy may be used if a person is exposed to another person with plague or an animal suspected of having plague.

A human vaccine is available for people who are at high risk, but it is not available in the United States. It does not protect people from pneumonic plague.

PSITTACOSIS

Psittacosis is a bacterial disease transmitted from bird to bird and from birds to humans. It is also known as *ornithosis*, *parrot fever*, *chlamydophilosis*, and *chlamydiosis* (not the sexually transmitted chlamydiosis).

MORBIDITY: +
MORTALITY: ++
ETIOLOGY: BACTERIAL

Psittacosis is caused by *Chlamydophila psittaci* (formerly *Chlamydia psittaci*), a coccoid, gram-negative, obligate intracellular (it must be inside a cell to reproduce) bacterium. *C. psittaci* can survive, and stay infective, outside of a host in the environment for several months.

HOSTS

The reservoir hosts for *C. psittaci* are pet birds, especially psittacine birds (such as parrots, parakeets, cockatiels, and macaws) from tropical and subtropical regions, and pigeons. *C. psittaci* has also been found in mynah birds, doves, canaries, birds of prey, shore birds, and domestic turkeys and ducks but only rarely in chickens. It has been found in more than 100 species of birds, but the most common sources of infection for people are pet psittacine birds and domestic turkeys.

TRANSMISSION

Transmission of *C. psittaci* is usually by inhalation. The organism is shed in fecal and nasal discharges of infected birds. When these discharges, especially the feces, dry, *C. psittaci* becomes airborne on fine, dried particles that can be inhaled by people or other birds. Other means of transmission include handling the plumage of infected birds and beak-to-mouth transmission. For this reason, owners should not kiss their pet birds. Rarely, a person with psittacosis may transmit *C. psittaci* to another person through violent, uncontrolled coughing.

PSITTACOSIS IN BIRDS

Psittacosis is highly contagious among birds. Some birds with psittacosis can shed *C. psittaci* but show no signs of disease. Stress is an important factor in birds developing clinical signs of psittacosis. Poor diet, overcrowding, poor sanitation, shipping, chilling, breeding, and relocation are some of the more important stressors that can cause a latent illness. In a latent illness, the bird has a *C. psittaci* infection, but shows no clinical sign of the disease until it is stressed. It may or may not be shedding *C. psittaci* during the latent period, which may last several years.

The incubation period between exposure to *C. psittaci* and the appearance of clinical signs is 3 days to several weeks. When clinical signs appear, they can include lethargy and depression, ruffled feathers with shivering, anorexia, ocular and nasal discharges, respiratory distress, diarrhea, yellowish to dark green droppings, decreased egg production, emaciation, and death.

PSITTACOSIS IN HUMANS

People at risk for developing psittacosis are those who are exposed to birds, such as pet shop employees, pet bird owners, veterinarians and veterinary technicians, farmers, wildlife rehabilitators, zoo workers, and workers in poultry slaughterhouses. Even casual exposure to birds can result in infection. Infected people frequently acquire the *C. psittaci* infection by inhaling dust from dried droppings in birdcages. The incubation period, from exposure to clinical illness, is 4 to 15 days.

Psittacosis is primarily a lung disease. It begins with flulike symptoms that include fever, chills, headache, lethargy, sensitivity to light, and anorexia. A nonproductive cough that is accompanied by difficult breathing and tightness in the chest may develop. Severe pneumonia that will require hospitalization and intensive, supportive care may also develop.

Occasionally the infection spreads beyond the lungs to affect the heart, liver, kidney, or brain. When this happens, hepatitis, endocarditis, and neurological signs may develop that require more intensive, supportive therapy.

The fever will last 2 to 3 weeks. Without treatment, uncomplicated psittacosis can be fatal; with treatment it rarely is.

DIAGNOSIS

Diagnosis in birds can be based on clinical signs and serologic testing. A positive serologic test result indicates that the bird was infected with *C. psittaci* at some point but does not confirm that the bird has an active infection.

In people, diagnosis begins with a history of exposure to birds, their plumage, or dried discharges. The clinical signs are nonspecific, but the respiratory involvement should point to psittacosis. Serologic testing can be helpful in establishing a diagnosis, but some tests are not highly specific. *C. psittaci* may be found in a patient's sputum, fluid from the thorax, or blood at the beginning of the infection, but culturing the organism is difficult and dangerous, so very few laboratories will do it.

Human cases of psittacosis must be reported to state public health officials.

TREATMENT

In birds treatment must last 45 days. Specific antibiotics can be given in food, water, orally, or by intramuscular injection. There is no guarantee that the infection will be completely eliminated with this treatment protocol, but many birds are returned to normal health if treatment is continued for the entire 45 days.

Treatment for psittacosis in people involves specific antibiotics. They are usually administered orally, but can also be given intravenously in severe cases. Treatment must continue for at least 2 weeks after the fever is gone. When treated most people recover without incident. Without treatment, the disease may become severe or fatal. Children and pregnant women require alternative drug therapy.

PREVENTION

There is no vaccine available for psittacosis. Prevention in birds and people involves minimizing exposure to *C. psittaci*:

- Keep stress in birds as low as possible to prevent any latent diseases from developing. This will help minimize *C. psittaci* shedding in the feces.
- Sick birds should be isolated from healthy birds to prevent spread.
- On the advice of a veterinarian, healthy birds may be put on medicated feed or water as a prophylactic measure.
- Keep birds and bird cages clean to prevent buildup of dried fecal material.
- Imported psittacine birds must be quarantined when entering the United States. During the quarantine period, they are given antibiotics to help prevent psittacosis. Buying illegally imported birds increases the risk of *C. psittaci* infection.
- In a pet shop or any flock situation, newly arrived birds should be isolated from resident birds.
- Keep circulation of dust and feathers at a minimum. When cleaning rooms where birds are kept, moisten the floor first with a disinfectant solution.

Wear a face mask when cleaning cages and floors. Clean the cages with a disinfectant solution. A 1:100 household bleach solution, made by adding 2 tablespoons of bleach to a gallon of water, works well. Lysol, Roccal-D, or Zephiran solutions also are effective disinfectants. Follow the disinfectant with a wash of warm, soapy water and a clean water rinse.

- Clean cages and rooms where sick birds are kept *after* cleaning cages or rooms where healthy birds are kept. This will help prevent accidental spread of psittacosis from sick birds to healthy birds.

Q FEVER

Q fever can be a chronic, debilitating, possibly fatal infection. It is transmitted to humans through contact with infected reproductive tissues, especially the birthing fluids and placenta, of cattle, sheep, and goats. "Q" is for "query," because the people who first recognized the disease did not know what caused it.

MORBIDITY: +
MORTALITY: +
ETIOLOGY: BACTERIAL

Coxiella burnetii is responsible for Q fever in people and animals. *C. burnetii* is a small, gram-negative coccobacillus that lives and multiplies in the monocytes and macrophages in the host. As the organism multiplies, it destroys the host cell and moves on to live in other cells. Q fever is unique in that it does not require a tick bite to transfer the bacteria from host to host, although tick bite transmission has been seen in animals. *C. burnetii* can survive outside of a host in the environment for weeks to months. A single *C. burnetii* organism can cause disease.

HOSTS

Cattle, sheep, and goats are the most common reservoirs of *C. burnetii*. It has also been found in dogs and cats. Some ticks have been shown to carry *C. burnetii*.

TRANSMISSION

C. burnetii is shed primarily in the birthing fluids of cattle, sheep, and goats. It is also found in milk, urine, and feces and is transmitted to people and other animals through inhalation of *C. burnetii* in fine-particle aerosols. Rarely, transmission can occur from ingestion of contaminated, unpasteurized milk or other dairy products. Contaminated bedding materials, such as straw used as packing materials, can transmit Q fever long distances.

Q FEVER IN ANIMALS

Animals are primarily asymptomatic carriers that act as reservoirs of *C. burnetii* for people and other animals. Rarely, abortion, still births, and difficult deliveries may occur in infected ruminants.

Q FEVER IN HUMANS

Q fever in humans is mostly an occupational hazard for people who may be exposed to aerosolized *C. burnetii* from birthing fluids. This group includes veterinarians, veterinary technicians, livestock farmers, dairy workers, slaughterhouse workers, and researchers at facilities where ruminants are housed. *C. burnetii* infection in people results in clinical illness in about half of the people who become infected. Clinical signs appear 1 to 3 weeks following infection, and the disease initially presents like the flu, with fever, sore throat, chills, headache, lethargy, muscle pains, nausea, vomiting, diarrhea, night sweats, and abdominal or chest pains. Some people will develop mental confusion, hepatitis, or *endocarditis*, inflammation of the lining of the heart. About a third of the patients showing clinical signs will develop pneumonia. The fever can last up to 2 weeks, and without treatment, the patient may recover to normal health over several months.

If the infection lasts over 6 months, or reappears after apparent recovery, it is considered chronic Q fever. Fewer than 5% of people who have acute Q fever will develop chronic Q fever. Sometimes a person recovers from acute Q fever only to develop the signs of chronic Q fever up to 20 years later.

The most significant sign of chronic Q fever is endocarditis, which may affect the heart valves. Hepatitis and arthritis are also sometimes seen with chronic Q fever.

DIAGNOSIS

In humans, Q fever is diagnosed using serologic tests to detect antibodies against *C. burnetii*. A history of exposure to birthing fluids and tissues may help in establishing an initial diagnosis, but the clinical signs of acute Q fever are too nonspecific to be diagnostic.

In animals, serologic testing is not as useful for diagnosis, because high serum antibodies can mean the animal has been exposed to *C. burnetii*, but they do not necessarily mean the animal is a current source of infection to other animals or people.

Serologic tests performed on a pooled milk sample is used to detect *C. burnetii* infection within a herd.

TREATMENT

In humans, treatment consists of long-term therapy including antibiotics and antimalarial drugs. Some patients will recover without treatment.

Treatment in animals is questionable because most animals are asymptomatic. If *C. burnetii* infection is known to exist in a herd, an antibiotic may be put in the water for several weeks before the beginning of the birthing season to decrease the number of *C. burnetii* organisms in the placenta and birthing fluids.

PREVENTION

No vaccine against *C. burnetii* infection is commercially available in the United States.

The best prevention in people is to reduce possible exposure to infected tissues and fluids. This includes properly disposing of all birthing products and aborted fetuses, disinfecting birthing areas if possible, consuming only pasteurized milk and dairy products, educating at-risk people about the signs of Q fever, and encouraging them to seek medical treatment as soon as possible if they think they are infected.

In animals, minimizing their exposure to birthing tissues and fluids through proper disposal and sanitation is the best prevention.

RABIES

Rabies is probably one of the best known and deadliest zoonotic diseases in the world. It has been around for thousands of years and strikes fear in people everywhere.

MORBIDITY: +
MORTALITY: ++++
ETIOLOGY: VIRAL

Infection with the rabies virus results in acute encephalitis in most mammals, including humans. Without treatment before signs and symptoms appear, the outcome is almost always fatal.

HOSTS

The vast majority of rabies cases reported to the CDC each year occur in wild animals such as raccoons, skunks, bats, and foxes. Domestic animals account for less than 10% of reported rabies cases, with cats, cattle, and dogs most often affected. Although all species of mammals are susceptible to rabies virus infection, only a few species are important as reservoirs for the disease.

In North America, several distinct rabies virus variants have been identified in terrestrial mammals, including raccoons, skunks, foxes, and coyotes. In addition to these terrestrial reservoirs, several species of insectivorous bats are also reservoirs for rabies. Rodents and lagomorphs, like rabbits and hares, are unlikely to have rabies.

TRANSMISSION

Various routes of transmission have been documented and include bites, contamination of mucous membranes, aerosol transmission, and organ and tissue transplants. The most common mode of rabies virus transmission is through a bite wound contaminated with virus-containing saliva from an infected animal. The virus cannot penetrate intact skin. Under refrigeration or during colder winter months, the virus can live from 4 weeks up to several months in dead animals. The virus will no longer be infective after a couple of hours in dried blood or other secretions.

THE DISEASE

Following infection, the virus enters an eclipse phase, during which it cannot be easily detected within the host. During the eclipse phase, the host's immune defenses may stimulate a cell-mediated immunity against the rabies virus antigen. About 20% of people exposed to the virus develop rabies when the cell-mediated immunity does not neutralize the virus.

The uptake of virus into peripheral nerves is important for infection to occur. After uptake into peripheral nerves, the rabies virus is transported to the central nervous system. Typically this occurs by way of the sensory and motor nerves at the initial site of infection.

The incubation period may vary, from a few days to several years, but is typically 1 to 3 months. There is a direct relationship between the location of the bite and the length of the incubation period. Bites on the head, neck, and arms progress most quickly, because of the close proximity of the central nervous system to these locations. The amount of virus received is also significant. A bite through clothing may result in some of the saliva being absorbed by the clothing, which could reduce the number of viruses that enter the bite wound.

The virus spreads rapidly within the central nervous system. Active cerebral infection is followed by spread of the virus back to the peripheral nerves. This may lead to viral invasion of highly innervated sites, including the salivary glands.

RABIES IN ANIMALS

During the period of cerebral infection, the classic behavioral changes associated with rabies develop. Rabid animals of all species exhibit signs typical of central nervous system disturbance.

The clinical course, particularly in dogs, can be divided into three phases: the *prodromal*, the *excitative*, and the *paralytic*. The term *furious rabies* refers to cases in which the *excitative phase* is predominant. *Dumb* or *paralytic rabies* refers to cases in which the excitative phase is short or absent. The disease progresses quickly to the *paralytic phase*, characterized by flaccid paralysis that leads to eventual death due to respiratory and/or cardiac failure.

In any animal, the first clinical signs of rabies are seen in the *prodromal stage*. These signs can include a change in behavior, which may be indistinguishable from a variety of other disorders, such as gastrointestinal disorder, injury, a foreign body in the mouth, poisoning, or an early infectious disease. Body temperature change is not significant, and slobbering may or may not be noted. Animals usually stop eating and drinking and may seek solitude. Frequently, the urogenital tract is irritated or stimulated, resulting in frequent urination, erection in the male, and signs of increased sexual desire.

After the prodromal period of 2 to 4 days, animals either become vicious or show signs of paralysis. Carnivores, pigs, and occasionally horses and mules bite other animals or people at the slightest provocation. Cattle may butt any moving object. Rabid domestic cats and bobcats attack suddenly, biting and scratching viciously. Rabid foxes frequently invade yards or even houses, attacking dogs and people. Rabid foxes and skunks are responsible for most pasture cattle losses from rabies and have even attacked cattle in barns.

A rabid raccoon is characterized by a loss of fear of humans, frequent aggression and incoordination, and abnormal activity during the day (raccoons are predominantly nocturnal animals). In urban areas, rabid skunks and raccoons often attack domestic dogs. Skunks are the leading reservoir of rabies in large areas of the United States. Bats flying in daytime are probably rabid.

The disease progresses rapidly after the onset of paralysis, and death is virtually certain within 10 days of the first clinical signs.

RABIES IN HUMANS

The first signs and symptoms of human rabies may be flulike and include malaise, fever, or headache, which may last for days. There may be discomfort or tingling at the site of initial exposure, developing within days to symptoms of cerebral dysfunction, anxiety, confusion, and agitation, progressing to delirium, abnormal behavior, hallucinations, and insomnia. Attempts at drinking cause extremely painful laryngeal spasms, so that the patient refuses to drink. This leads to the historical name for rabies, *hydrophobia*.

Several factors may affect the outcome of rabies exposure. These include the virus variant, the dose of virus received, and the type and location of exposure, as well as individual host factors, such as age and immune defenses.

Although rabies among humans is rare in the United States, every year an estimated 18,000 people receive rabies preexposure prophylaxis, and an additional 40,000 receive postexposure prophylaxis.

DIAGNOSIS

Several tests are necessary to diagnose rabies *antemortem*, or before death, in humans; no single test is sufficient. Saliva, serum, skin biopsy specimens, and spinal fluid can be tested for various indicators of the presence of the rabies virus.

The standard test for rabies is a postmortem test, based on the presence of rabies virus protein, or *antigen*, in nervous tissue, especially the brain. Other diagnostic tests are also available.

Animals with a current rabies vaccination history may be quarantined for observation for 10 days after biting a human, to see if clinical signs of rabies appear. Animals with an unknown rabies vaccination history are euthanized immediately after biting a human. The brains of these animals are examined for rabies antigen.

A thorough history of the bite event is critical.

TREATMENT

Once clinical signs of rabies appear, the disease is nearly always fatal, and treatment is typically supportive.

There is no sanctioned treatment for rabies after signs and symptoms of the disease appear. However, there is an extremely effective rabies vaccine regimen that provides immunity to rabies when administered after an exposure or for protection before an exposure occurs.

Treatment of a person who has been exposed to the rabies virus is entirely prophylactic, so postexposure prophylaxis includes both immune globulin (passive antibody) and vaccine. To date, only six documented cases of human survival from clinical rabies have been reported.

PRE-EXPOSURE VACCINATION

Pre-exposure vaccination is recommended for persons in high-risk groups, such as veterinary technicians, veterinarians, animal handlers, and some laboratory workers. Other people whose activities bring them into frequent contact with the rabies virus or potentially rabid bats, raccoons, skunks, cats, dogs, or other species at risk of having rabies should also consider pre-exposure vaccination. In addition, international travelers likely to come in contact with animals in areas of enzootic dog rabies and who lack immediate access to appropriate medical care also should consider pre-exposure vaccination.

The purpose of pre-exposure vaccinations is to protect the recipients against the full effects of the rabies virus if they are exposed to the virus. Although pre-exposure vaccination does not eliminate the need for additional medical attention after rabies virus exposure, it simplifies therapy by eliminating the need for human rabies immune globulin (RIG) and decreasing the number of postexposure vaccine doses needed. Pre-exposure vaccination consists of three intramuscular doses of rabies vaccine, given on day 0 (the day of the first vaccine injection), day 7, and either day 21 or day 28. The effectiveness of the preexposure vaccination is measured by checking the recipient's blood titer (amount of antibodies present) on a regular basis. If the titer gets too low, the vaccine is readministered.

POSTEXPOSURE PROPHYLAXIS

Postexposure prophylaxis (PEP) is indicated for anyone who has possibly been exposed to a rabid animal. Possible exposures include animal bites or mucous membrane contamination with infectious tissue, such as saliva. PEP should begin as soon as possible after an exposure. There have been no vaccine failures in the United States when PEP was given as soon as possible and appropriately after an exposure.

Administration of PEP is a medical urgency, not a medical emergency. Physicians evaluate each possible exposure to rabies and may consult with local or state public health officials regarding the need for rabies prophylaxis.

In the United States, PEP consists of a regimen of one dose of human RIG (approximately half of the dose is infused around the wound, with the rest administered intramuscularly at some point distant from it) and five doses of human diploid cell vaccine (HDCV; a rabies vaccine made from a specific cell culture of human cells) over a 28-day period. The vaccine is given as five intramuscular injections, at day 0 (the day of the first injection), day 3, day 7, day 14, and day 28 after exposure. RIG and the first dose of HDCV should be given as soon as possible after exposure. The injections are no longer given in the abdominal area, where they were very painful.

If you are exposed to a potentially rabid animal, wash the wound thoroughly with soap and water, encourage bleeding from the wound, and seek medical attention immediately. The following information will help the health care provider assess risk:
• The geographic location of the incident
• The type of animal involved
• How the exposure occurred (provoked or unprovoked)
• The vaccination status of the animal
• Whether the animal can be captured safely and observed or tested for rabies

PREVENTION

People need to be responsible animal owners. Rabies vaccinations should be kept up-to-date for all dogs, cats, and ferrets. This is important, not only to keep pets from getting rabies, but also to provide a barrier of protection for owners, veterinary and medical personnel, and anyone else who comes in contact with animals bitten by a rabid wild animal. Each state determines how often rabies vaccine must be administered to animals living in that state. The following are ways to minimize the risk of exposure to rabies:

- Spaying and neutering pets helps reduce the number of unwanted pets that may not be properly cared for or regularly vaccinated.
- Avoid direct contact with unfamiliar animals, including stray animals. Calls about stray animals should be referred to the local animal control agency so the animals can be removed from the neighborhood. These animals may be unvaccinated and could be infected with the rabies virus. Teach children never to approach or handle unfamiliar animals, wild or domestic, even if they appear friendly. "Love your own; leave others alone" is a good principle for children to learn.
- Pet owners should keep their pets under direct supervision so they do not come in contact with wild animals. Enjoy wild animals from afar.
- Do not handle, feed, or unintentionally attract wild animals with open garbage cans or litter. Never adopt wild animals or bring them into homes.
- Prevent bats from entering living quarters or occupied spaces in homes, churches, schools, and other similar areas, where they might come in contact with people and pets.
- When traveling abroad, avoid direct contact with animals. Be especially careful around dogs in developing countries, where rabies control or immediate medical treatment might not be available.

HISTORICAL NOTE

Rabies has been known as a lethal, infectious disease of the central nervous system as far back as 2300 BC. Before 1885 a bite from a rabid animal meant certain death. On July 6, 1885, Louis Pasteur heralded the modern era of immunization when he injected the first of 14 daily doses of rabbit spinal cord suspensions containing progressively inactivated rabies virus into Joseph Meister, a 9-year-old boy who had been bitten by a rabid dog 2 days earlier. Joseph made a total recovery and remained healthy for the rest of his life. He returned to the Pasteur Institute as an employee, where he served for many years as gatekeeper.

In 1940, 55 years after his treatment for rabies that made medical history, and 45 years after Louis Pasteur died, Joseph was ordered by the German occupiers of Paris to open Pasteur's crypt. Rather than comply, he committed suicide!*

---

*From a lecture presented by David V. Cohn, School of Dentistry, University of Louisville, Feb. 11, 1996.

RAT-BITE FEVER

Rat-bite fever (RBF) is an uncommon bacterial infection that results from exposure to infected rodents, usually through a bite or scratch wound. It is also known as *Haverhill fever*, *streptobacillary fever*, and *epidemic arthritic erythema*.

MORBIDITY: +

MORTALITY: +

ETIOLOGY: BACTERIAL

RBF is caused by *Streptobacillus moniliformis*, a gram-negative bacillus.

HOSTS

S. moniliformis is found in the mouth, nasopharynx, nasal and ocular discharges, feces, and urine of laboratory and wild rodents. It has also been found in pet rats. All appear to be healthy carriers.

TRANSMISSION

RBF is transmitted to people from the mouth of an infected rodent through a bite or scratch wound; through ingestion of food, water, or milk contaminated with feces or urine; or through contact with ocular or nasal discharges of an infected rat. RBF is not transmitted from person to person.

RAT-BITE FEVER IN ANIMALS

Wild and laboratory rodents appear to be reservoirs of *S. moniliformis*, but are not affected by the organism. Immunodeficient mice and rats may develop polyarthritis, gangrene, and loss of limbs.

RAT-BITE FEVER IN HUMANS

Clinical signs of RBF appear 2 to 10 days after exposure to *S. moniliformis*. By this time the original bite wound, if one was present, has healed. RBF begins with an acute fever and chills, followed by flulike symptoms including nausea, vomiting, lethargy, headache, joint pain, back pain, and muscle pain. In another 2 to 4 days, a rash of tiny red bumps appears on the palms of the hands and soles of the feet, and some larger joints become inflamed.

People most susceptible to *S. moniliformis* infection are those who work in laboratories or people in poor living conditions, where rat infestations are more prevalent. Children living in poor conditions are especially susceptible to RBF because they are more often bitten. Infected pet rats can transmit *S. moniliformis* through bites or scratches.

If RBF is not treated, serious complications such as heart valve infection, endocarditis, pericarditis, pneumonia, meningitis, or organ abscesses may result.

DIAGNOSIS

Initial diagnosis is based on a history of rodent exposure and clinical signs. Blood or joint fluid can be cultured, but *S. moniliformis* is difficult to grow. Noninfected rats can be inoculated with fluid from an infected person to see if infection develops. Serologic tests can detect the presence of *S. moniliformis* antibodies in infected people.

TREATMENT

Thoroughly clean any wound or scratch from a rodent. It is important to scrub the wound several times, over a period of several minutes, using soap under warm, running water. Use a scrub brush if one is available; this will get rid of as much of the bacteria as possible. Follow the scrubbing with an antiseptic solution, such as iodine or Betadine (povidone-iodine solution).

Antibiotic therapy is administered to prevent serious, possibly fatal, complications.

A tetanus booster should be given if the patient is not currently protected.

PREVENTION

There is no vaccine available to protect against RBF. Follow these safeguards to minimize exposure:

- Avoid contact with wild rats or rat-contaminated environments.
- Do not eat food or drink water or milk that may be contaminated with rat feces or urine.
- Wear gloves and protective clothing when working with rats or other rodents in a laboratory.
- After handling rodents, wash hands thoroughly.
- Take time to thoroughly cleanse every wound or scratch from a rat or other rodent.

ROCKY MOUNTAIN SPOTTED FEVER

Rocky Mountain spotted fever (RMSF) is the most severe and most commonly reported tick-borne rickettsial disease in the United States. RMSF has been reported in every state but occurs more frequently in the south-Atlantic states. There are numerous "spotted" diseases, caused by different species of *Rickettsia*, but only RMSF occurs in the United States.

MORBIDITY: +
MORTALITY: +
ETIOLOGY: BACTERIAL

Rickettsia rickettsii is the bacterium responsible for causing RMSF in people. It is a gram-negative, obligate intracellular bacterium. In the case of RMSF, the cells invaded initially are the cells that line small- to medium-size blood vessels. When *R. rickettsii* multiplies, it kills the cells, causing blood to leak out of the vessels into the surrounding tissue. Since blood vessels are virtually everywhere in the body, *R. rickettsii* can cause blood seepage into just about any tissue. This makes RMSF a potential multiorgan disease. The leakage also causes a rash, or *spotted fever*, to develop in 85% to 90% of people who become ill.

HOSTS

Ticks are both reservoirs and vectors for RMSF. Hard, or *ixodid*, ticks spread the disease to humans. So far the American dog tick (*Dermacentor variabilis*) and the Rocky Mountain wood tick (*Dermacentor andersoni*) are the most common culprits in the United States. The brown dog tick (*Rhipicephalus sanguineus*), which transmits RMSF more commonly in Mexico, has been implicated in an RMSF outbreak in Arizona. These ticks do not feed exclusively on people, so *R. rickettsii* is found in many vertebrates.

TRANSMISSION

People are infected primarily by the bite of a tick. Rarely, people become infected by crushing an infected tick with their fingers, allowing tick fluids to enter through cuts or broken skin.

The tick life cycle has three active stages after the egg hatches: larva, nymph, and adult (Appendix 1). The larva must have a blood meal before it can molt to the nymph stage, and the nymph must have a blood meal before it can molt to the adult stage. The tick becomes infected when it takes blood from an infected animal or person. The bacteria stay with the tick when it molts to the next stage. As it feeds before molting, and at any stage, it can infect another animal or person by depositing *R. rickettsii* when it bites. Ticks in all three stages feed on people. A tick needs to be attached to a person for at least 6 hours before *R. rickettsii* is transmitted (Figure 30).

Once infected, a tick can carry *R. rickettsii* for its entire life. Female ticks can also become infected when male ticks transmit the organism through body fluids or spermatozoa. The female tick can pass *R. rickettsii* to her eggs through transovarian transmission.

ROCKY MOUNTAIN SPOTTED FEVER IN ANIMALS

Ticks that are infected with *R. rickettsii* remain healthy. Dogs are the only nonhuman animal that will show clinical signs of RMSF. The clinical signs are similar to those found in humans.

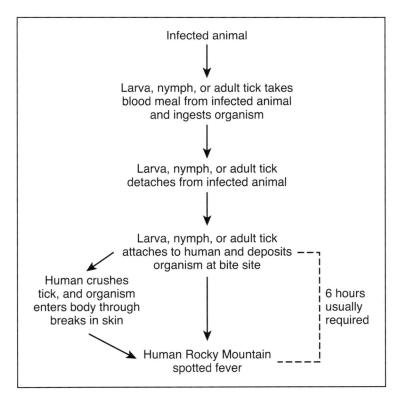

FIGURE 30.   Rocky Mountain spotted fever.

ROCKY MOUNTAIN SPOTTED FEVER IN HUMANS

In people, RMSF develops about 5 to 10 days after a tick bite. Many times people do not even remember being bitten. The early signs are not specific for RMSF and may include fever, chills, muscle aches, and headache. Nausea, vomiting, anorexia, lethargy, edema in the extremities, and swollen joints may also be seen. About 2 to 5 days after the fever develops, a rash appears in 85% to 90% of the patients showing clinical signs (Figure 31). The rash begins as nonitchy, flat, pink spots on the wrists, forearms, palms, ankles, and soles. The spots are called *macules*. From there, they spread toward the trunk; the face is spared in most cases. When pressed, the spots blanch (turn white). Eventually they turn dark red and disappear without leaving a scar.

People who do not develop the rash are said to have Rocky Mountain *spotless* fever. These people tend to suffer more severe forms of the disease.

As RMSF develops, organ and tissue damage begins. This happens rapidly. Many people will be so severely affected that they will require hospitalization. The systems most often affected are the central nervous system, respiratory system, renal system, hepatic system, and gastrointestinal tract. Clinical signs will vary depending on which systems are affected.

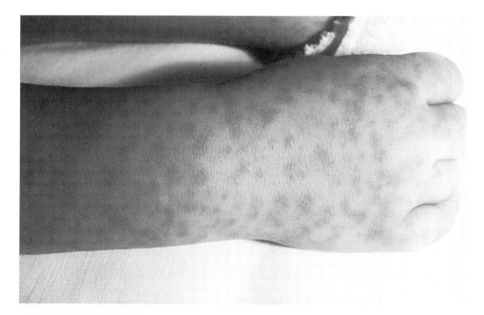

FIGURE 31.   Rocky Mountain spotted fever in a human. (Courtesy Public Health Image Library, PHIL 1962, Centers for Disease Control and Prevention, Atlanta.)

Long-term complications may follow an acute case of RMSF. They include partial paralysis; hearing loss; loss of bladder or bowel control; or gangrene that may lead to amputation of fingers, toes, arms, or legs. These complications are most often seen in patients who have survived a more severe case of RMSF and have been hospitalized for a long time.

DIAGNOSIS

When diagnosing RMSF, physicians or veterinarians look for what they call the *triad of clinical findings*, which includes fever, rash, and a history of tick bite. The rash may not have developed when the patient first seeks medical help, so often the fever and a history of a tick bite are the bases of diagnosis. If a person does not remember being bitten by a tick, RMSF may go undiagnosed during an initial examination. This could also be the case for some dogs, in which a tick that would aid diagnosis is not found.

Serologic testing can confirm a diagnosis, but it is based on finding the antibodies against *R. rickettsii* in two separate blood samples taken after the patient begins to recover.

TREATMENT

Treatment must begin as soon as possible to be effective. Appropriate antibiotics are available. The sooner treatment begins, the lower the mortality rate. After 5 days without treatment, the mortality rate triples, and older patients are twice as likely to die as younger ones. Treatment cannot wait until laboratory tests confirm RMSF.

PREVENTION

There is no vaccine available to protect against RMSF. The best prevention is to avoid areas where ticks are most active during the months when they are prevalent, typically April through September. When entering tick-infested areas, the following steps will help decrease exposure (Appendix 2):

- Avoid areas where ticks thrive as much as possible. April through September are the months when ticks are most active.
- Wear light-colored clothing when entering an area that may be a habitat for ticks. This will make the adult ticks easier to see and remove before they become attached.
- Wear long-sleeved shirts and long pants tucked into socks so the ticks cannot crawl under clothing; wear high rubber boots and a hat for the same reason.

- Walk in the center of trails to avoid vegetation where ticks are lurking. Ticks cannot fly, jump, skip, or hop, so they must come in direct contact with a host before they can attach themselves. Immature ticks are found hiding in the shade in moist areas. Adult ticks cling to grass, bushes, and shrubs, waiting for a host to come by.
- Exposed skin and clothing can be protected with insect repellents containing DEET. These repellents must be reapplied every few hours. Clothes, but not exposed skin, can be protected with insect repellents containing permethrin, which kills ticks on contact. These repellents stay on clothes for several days.
- Check often for ticks while outside.
- Do not sit on the ground.
- Make daily checks of the entire body for ticks. Look especially in areas where ticks like to attach, such as behind the ears, at the back of the neck, in the armpits, behind the knees, and in the groin area. Bathing will remove crawling ticks but will not detach ticks already attached.
- Wash and dry outdoor clothing after use using high temperatures.
- Remove ticks as soon as they are found. Remember, it takes 6 hours after a tick becomes attached before it starts releasing *R. rickettsii*.
- To remove the tick, use fine tweezers; grasp the tick as close to the skin as possible, and pull straight back, with slow, steady force. Avoid crushing the tick's body. Kill the tick by dropping it in alcohol; save the tick in alcohol as a possible diagnostic aid.
- Ticks can be carried into a home by pets, so check them often and thoroughly if they have been in tick-infested areas. Use tick collars or other medications to prevent ticks from attaching to pets.
- Ticks can also transmit RSMF to dogs, so it is especially important that dogs be checked thoroughly and often for ticks.

ROUNDWORMS

Roundworms belong to the phylum Nematoda, which contains worms that are round and unsegmented. Members of this phylum are called *nematodes*. There are thousands of genera of nematodes, but only five are of zoonotic importance in North America: *Toxocara canis, T. cati, Baylisascaris procyonis, Ancylostoma braziliense, and Trichinella spp*. *A. braziliense* is a nematode parasite that is discussed under Hookworms. *Trichinella spp*. are discussed under trichinosis.

MORBIDITY: +
MORTALITY: + TO ++++
ETIOLOGY: PARASITIC

T. canis, T. cati, and *B. procyonis* are roundworms of zoonotic importance when the infective eggs of these parasites are ingested by abnormal, or atypical, *dead-end* mammalian hosts, such as people.

HOSTS

T. canis is the roundworm of dogs, *T. cati* is the roundworm of cats, and *B. procyonis* is the roundworm of raccoons. Other mammals, including humans, are abnormal or suboptimal hosts.

TRANSMISSION

Adult roundworms live in the intestines of their hosts. Transmission starts with passage of roundworm eggs in the feces. A single *T. canis* female can produce up to 100,000 eggs per day; a single *B. procyonis* female can produce up to 45,000,000 eggs per day. If the host is harboring hundreds of roundworms, the potential exists for the production of millions of infective eggs in a single day. Roundworm eggs can become infective within 2 weeks and can remain infective in the environment for years. Eggs often live in soil, and the next host is infected when it eats infective eggs containing live larvae or immature worms.

After ingestion the eggs hatch, and the larvae are released into the intestinal tract. They burrow through the intestinal wall and into a blood vessel, where they are then carried on a circuitous journey through the host's body. Eventually they end up back in the host's intestines when they are ready to become adults. The cycle begins again after the adult female roundworms produce eggs, which are then passed in the host's feces (Figure 31).

The zoonotic problem arises when the infective roundworm eggs are ingested by atypical or suboptimal hosts, such as people. The eggs still hatch in the intestine, and the larvae will enter the blood stream to begin migration routes that are abnormal because the larvae are in an atypical host. These abnormal migration routes do not lead back to the intestines, but along the way the larvae are deposited in various tissues in the body, causing tissue damage as they continue to migrate through the tissue.

ROUNDWORM INFECTIONS IN ANIMALS

Damage due to roundworms is most often seen in young animals. Puppies can be infected with *T. canis* before they are born, through the mother's milk, or by ingesting infective eggs. Sometimes migrating larvae in a bitch will go dormant in tissue until she becomes pregnant. If she has been treated for roundworms, she most likely is not shedding roundworm eggs in the feces, so she appears to be roundworm-free. The pregnancy activates the larvae to finish the life cycle, and they find their way back to the intestines, where they mature and produce eggs. Puppies can thus become infected from a mother that appears roundworm-free.

Kittens are not infected with *T. cati* before they are born, but are most likely to be infected through the mother's milk and through ingestion of infective eggs.

Adult worms absorb nutrients from the host's intestines. Because of their large size, they can interfere with digestion and may even damage the intestinal wall. In large numbers they can cause intestinal obstruction and constipation. Animals with low numbers of adult worms may show no roundworm-specific clinical signs. Puppies with heavy infections will be thin, but will have a potbelly. They may vomit or have diarrhea in which adult worms may be present. Adult worms may also be passed in the puppy's normal feces. Puppies with heavy infections do not do well, and often act as though they are in pain. *T. canis* and *T. cati* larvae migrate through the lungs, causing a dry cough.

The life cycle of *B. procyonis* is similar to the life cycles of *T. canis* and *T. cati*. The adult worms do not seem to do much damage in raccoons.

LARVA MIGRANS IN HUMANS

When people swallow roundworm eggs, they can develop diseases known as *visceral larval migrans, ocular larva migrans*, or *neural larva migrans* (Figure 32).

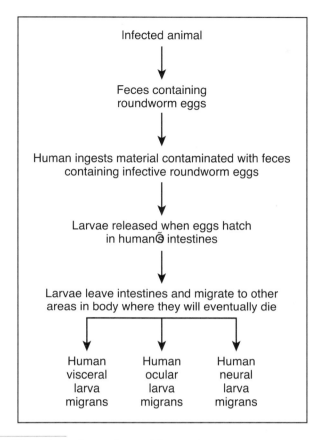

FIGURE 32.   Visceral, ocular, and neural larva migrans.

As with animals, most of the damage seen with *T. canis, T. cati*, or *B. procyonis* infection in people occurs in young children. Most infections happen when children play in areas contaminated with infective roundworm eggs. Children like to put interesting things in their mouths, including dirt, dirty toys, or dirty hands, all of which may have been contaminated with infective roundworm eggs. The eggs hatch as usual in the intestine, and the released larvae burrow through the intestine wall into the blood stream, which carries them to various parts of the body, depositing them in tissues. The larvae can remain alive for many weeks in the tissues, where they migrate around causing tissue damage and destruction. This is known as *visceral larva migrans (VLM)*. The tissues most often affected are the liver, lungs, eye, and brain. The damage caused by the migrating larvae is permanent and can result in severe visual, respiratory, or neurological conditions. The degree of damage or destruction is dependent on the number of larvae meandering through the tissue. Eventually the larvae die, and small abscesses or granulomas may form around them. In people, the larvae never fully mature.

People infected with few roundworm larvae may show no clinical signs because the tissue damage is minimal. The presence of clinical signs also depends on which tissues are affected. People with heavier infections of larvae will show clinical signs, based on which tissues are infected.

When the larvae travel to the eye they can cause inflammation and scarring of the retina, which can lead to permanent, partial blindness. This condition is known as *ocular larva migrans (OLM)*.

B. procyonis larvae are more harmful to people for two reasons. First, the *B. procyonis* larvae continue to grow as they migrate through the tissue, so they cause more tissue damage because of their larger size. Second, the *B. procyonis* larvae are more likely to migrate to the spinal cord and brain, causing neural larva migrans (NLM) (Figure 33). The NLM that results from *B. procyonis* larvae infection is often fatal. Even if a patient recovers there are lingering neurological problems including blindness, seizures, paralysis, mental retardation, and physical retardation.

Direct contact with dogs, cats, or raccoons that have roundworms cannot lead to infection, because roundworm eggs need to mature in soil before they become infective. One possible exception is *B. procyonis* eggs, which are covered with a sticky substance that may allow them to stick to the hair on a raccoon. If the eggs stay on the hair long enough to become infective, a person could become infected by handling the raccoon. Roundworm infection cannot be spread from person to person.

DIAGNOSIS

In dogs, cats, and raccoons, a definitive diagnosis of roundworm infection is based on finding roundworm eggs in feces during a microscopic examination. Sometimes diagnosis is based on seeing adult worms passed in feces or vomited material.

Serologic tests are available for diagnosis of *T. canis* larval infection in people. However, no serological test is widely available or commonly used for *B. procyonis* diagnosis. Diagnosis of *B. procyonis* infection is based on clinical signs and tissue biopsy. Tissue biopsy is tentative at best because the biopsy must include a cross-section of the larvae, which can be difficult to obtain.

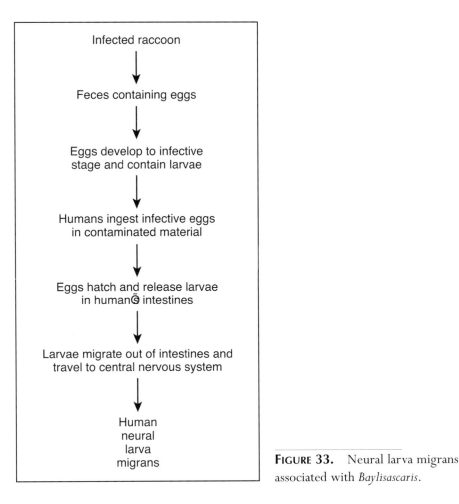

Infected raccoon

↓

Feces containing eggs

↓

Eggs develop to infective
stage and contain larvae

↓

Humans ingest infective eggs
in contaminated material

↓

Eggs hatch and release larvae
in humanⓈ intestines

↓

Larvae migrate out of intestines and
travel to central nervous system

↓

Human
neural
larva
migrans

FIGURE 33.   Neural larva migrans associated with *Baylisascaris*.

Even then there are other larvae that can be found in tissue, so the next hurdle is to confirm the identification of the larvae as *B. procyonis*.

TREATMENT

Dogs and cats are treated with antiparasitic drugs to rid them of roundworms. Raccoons, because they are wild animals, are not normally treated but could be if necessary.

In the case of *T. canis* or *T. cati*, VLM in people is treated with antiparasitic and antiinflammatory drugs. OLM is treated symptomatically to limit damage to the eye. There is no effective treatment for NLM caused by *B. procyonis*. NLM can result in sudden death or prolonged neurological problems for which there are no treatments.

PREVENTION

T. CANIS AND *T. CATI*

Prevention of roundworms in pets is based on eliminating the roundworms and controlling access to areas that are contaminated with roundworm eggs.

For pets this involves the following precautions:

- Deworm pets on a regular basis. Most veterinary clinics have a deworming protocol that includes treatment or prevention of roundworm infection.
- Puppies and kittens should be examined for roundworms and dewormed if necessary when they are very young. Again, most veterinary clinics will have a protocol for this, usually associated with the vaccination schedule.
- Keep areas where pets defecate clean. Feces should be removed at least once a week and disposed of where they will not come in contact with other animals and children. Feces can be buried or bagged and disposed of with the regular garbage.
- When away from home, limit the amount of contact your pet has with other animals or animal feces. Keep pets on a leash. With the advent of dog parks, this is becoming more difficult, especially if pet owners do not pick up after their dogs.

In people the following precautions can be taken:

- Keep pets free of roundworms.
- Do not allow children to play in areas that contain animal feces. Keep play areas, sandboxes, gardens, and lawns feces-free by regularly disposing of feces. Keep sandboxes covered when they are not in use. Watch children closely when they are in a dog park where animal feces may accumulate.
- Develop good sanitation habits when working or playing in areas where pet feces may accumulate. Flower beds, sandboxes, gardens, and lawns are areas where feces may lay long enough for the eggs to become infective. Always wash your hands and the hands of children after outdoor activities where animal feces may be present.
- Teach children why it could be dangerous to eat dirt.

SPECIAL *B. PROCYONIS* CONSIDERATIONS

With the spread of urbanization into normal rural raccoon habitats, it is important to understand some *B. procyonis* facts:

- The incidence of raccoon infection with *B. procyonis* is high. A raccoon can harbor many adult worms, and each female worm can shed as many as 45,000,000 eggs a day, for months or years.

- The eggs of *B. procyonis* are covered with a sticky substance that allows them to stick to fur and skin. A person could potentially become infected by handling a raccoon. Once the eggs are on the skin, the only practical way to remove them is to wash the skin with bleach. This removes the sticky substance, which will allow the eggs to fall off but does not kill them.
- Raccoons form latrine sites where they repeatedly defecate. In parks and wooded areas, these sites are commonly found on raised, horizontal surfaces such as stumps, logs, limbs, and forks or bases of trees. In urban and suburban areas, latrines also have been found in woodpiles; on roofs of houses, sheds, decks; and in sandboxes, patios, attics, chimneys, garages, and haylofts. A latrine site can be a source of infection for *B. procyonis*. Other sources are vegetation, bark, sand, and stones that have been contaminated with raccoon feces.
- It takes 3 to 4 weeks for *B. procyonis* eggs to become infective. By that time the fecal material is disintegrating and may be less obvious in the environment. *B. procyonis* eggs can survive for years in the environment and are resistant to heat, freezing, and all common disinfectants.
- *B. procyonis* eggs are difficult to kill. Bleach will remove the sticky substance on the surface of the eggs but will not kill the eggs. Extreme heat in the form of boiling water, steam, or a flame from a propane torch *will* kill the eggs. Wood, wood chips, or straw that may have contacted the eggs should be burned, not spread in other areas where contamination could occur.
- Where steam or fire are not practical, remove as much of the contaminated material as possible. On the ground, 2 to 3 inches (5 to 7.5 cm) of soil should be removed and discarded or burned. Do not put the soil where it could contaminate another area. If the latrine area was in a fireplace, remove the latrine and build a hot fire.

PREVENTING *B. PROCYONIS* INFECTION

- *Do not keep raccoons as pets!* Raccoons are wild animals. They also are susceptible to rabies infection.
- Avoid direct contact with raccoons and their feces. Do not feed them or encourage them to hang around.
- Discourage raccoons from living in and around your home or parks.
- Prevent access to food. Do not leave pet food or other foodstuffs unattended outside. Raccoons like the easy source of food.
- Close off access to attics, chimneys, and basements.

- Keep sandboxes covered at all times so they do not become latrines.
- Remove fish ponds. Raccoons eat the fish and drink the water.
- Eliminate easy-access water sources where raccoons may come to drink.
- Remove bird feeders. Raccoons eat seeds.
- Keep trash containers tightly closed to eliminate easy access to food.
- Clear brush so raccoons are not likely to make a den on your property.
- Stay away from areas and materials that might be contaminated by raccoon feces.

Decontaminate potentially contaminated areas appropriately, and remove latrines carefully. Wear protective clothing and footwear when working with or around raccoons or their latrines. Make sure the clothing and footwear are disposable or can withstand washing in boiling or near boiling water. If working around straw or wood, where there is a lot of dust, wear a dust mask.

ST. LOUIS ENCEPHALITIS

St. Louis encephalitis is a mosquito-borne viral disease with the potential of infecting the central nervous system of people. It is the most commonly reported variety of viral encephalitis in the United States, but is not nearly as common in Canada.

MORBIDITY: +
MORTALITY: + TO ++
ETIOLOGY: VIRAL

St. Louis encephalitis virus (SLEV) is an arbovirus (*arthropod-borne virus*) that causes St. Louis encephalitis (SLE). It is closely related to the West Nile virus. Other important encephalitis arboviruses include the eastern equine encephalitis virus, western equine encephalitis virus, and La Crosse encephalitis virus. SLEV was named for St. Louis, Missouri, where the first and largest epidemic occurred in 1933.

HOSTS

The natural hosts of SLEV are birds such as finches, sparrows, blue jays, cardinals, mockingbirds, blackbirds, robins, and doves.

TRANSMISSION

SLEV is passed from one bird to another by the bite of a mosquito. When a mosquito bites an infected bird, the virus replicates in the mosquito and moves to other locations in the mosquito's body, including the salivary glands. When the mosquito takes its next meal from an uninfected bird, it deposits a small drop of saliva where it bites to act as an anticoagulant. The saliva contains the virus, which enters the bird, replicates, and becomes a source of virus for other mosquitoes. Birds are considered *amplifiers* of SLEV, because one bird can potentially infect many mosquitoes (Figure 34).

Once a bird is infected, it replicates the virus for only a couple of days before the virus is eliminated. After that the bird becomes immune to further infection. As the number of immune birds increases, the number of birds that can pass the virus to mosquitoes decreases. This is one way nature controls outbreaks of SLE.

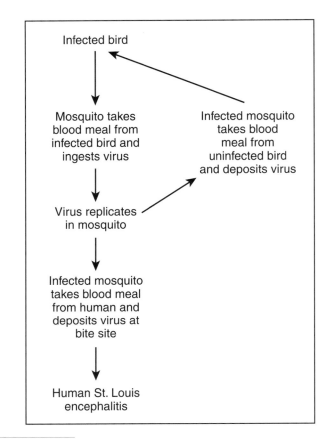

FIGURE 34.   St. Louis encephalitis.

Mosquitoes replicate the virus for their entire lives, but they live only a few days. Not all mosquitoes can transmit SLEV to people; only mosquitoes that feed on birds and mammals can transmit SLEV to people.

SLEV is transmitted to people by mosquitoes that have previously bitten infected birds. People are dead-end hosts; person-to-person transmission does not occur.

St. Louis Encephalitis in Animals

Birds and mosquitoes infected with SLEV do not develop any clinical signs of disease. No nonhuman animals seem to be affected.

ST. LOUIS ENCEPHALITIS IN HUMANS

Many people who become infected with SLEV do not develop clinical signs of illness. Once in a person's body, the virus is usually removed by macrophage cells, especially in the liver, spleen, and lymph nodes, which are filtering organs. Before clinical signs can develop, the virus level has to exceed the filtering capacity of these organs. In mild cases of SLE, people will show symptoms resembling the flu, including headache, fever, nausea, and vomiting.

In more severe cases, the virus can enter the central nervous system, resulting in encephalitis. The early signs are lethargy, fever, sore throat, and coughing; these are followed by headache, nausea, vomiting, confusion and disorientation, double vision, muscle tremors, neck stiffness, and spastic paralysis. Convulsions may occur in infants.

SLE is seen year-round in the southern United States and from late summer to early fall in the more temperate areas further north. The incubation period can be anywhere from 4 days to 3 weeks. People most at risk for developing SLE are the young, the elderly, people who live in crowded or unsanitary conditions, and people who work or play outdoors where SLE is common. Men are more commonly affected. The mortality rate is 3 to 30% and increases with the patient's age. People over 60 have the highest mortality rate. About 20% of survivors will have lingering memory loss, seizures, motor deficits, and irritability.

DIAGNOSIS

Diagnosis is based on the presence of antibodies against SLEV. The virus can be isolated from tissue, blood, or cerebral spinal fluid.

TREATMENT

As with most viral diseases, there is no specific drug to combat SLEV. Supportive care and management of neurological symptoms are the only treatments available.

PREVENTION

There is no vaccination available for protection against SLE in people. Prevention centers on decreased exposure to mosquitoes.

Reducing exposure to mosquitoes involves the following precautions:

- Drain areas of standing water, especially after rainfall or watering. These are mosquito breeding sites.
- Reduce outdoor activities during peak mosquito activity, from dusk to dawn.
- Wear protective clothing when mosquitoes are most active, especially in the early evening and early morning. Protective clothing includes long-sleeved shirts and long pants.
- Use insect repellent containing DEET on exposed skin.
- Make sure screens fit properly and are free from holes to decrease mosquito access to building interiors.

SALMONELLOSIS

Salmonellosis is a bacterial infection of the gastrointestinal tract that is usually associated with eating feces-contaminated food.

MORBIDITY: ++
MORTALITY: +
ETIOLOGY: BACTERIAL

Salmonellosis is caused by many serotypes of the *Salmonella* bacteria, which are gram-negative and *facultatively anaerobic*, meaning they live in the presence or absence of oxygen. *Salmonella* live in the intestinal tracts of people and animals; over 2000 serotypes have been identified. The two most common serotypes seen in the United States are *S. enteritidis* and *S. typhimurium* (causes typhoid fever, a human-only disease, so it will not be discussed here). Nontyphoidal salmonellosis is caused by *S. enteritidis* and results in the disease we associate with food poisoning. This serotype, and most others, are passed in the feces of an infected animal or person.

Some serotypes of *Salmonella* are species-specific and will not easily be spread to other species. Other serotypes are not species-specific, and these are the serotypes related to species-to-species spread, including the spread to people.

HOSTS

Salmonella resides in the intestinal tracts of both warm-blooded and cold-blooded animals. In people, anyone who is infected with the *Salmonella* organism can get sick, but it most commonly affects children under 5, elderly people, and people with compromised or weakened immune systems. Not every person or animal infected with *Salmonella* will become ill. *Salmonella* carriers often appear healthy.

TRANSMISSION

Many people become infected with *Salmonella* organisms by eating contaminated food, such as chicken, raw eggs, beef, milk, milk products, and vegetables (Figure 35). One outbreak of salmonellosis was caused by raw alfalfa sprouts, grown in contaminated soil. Any food of animal origin can be

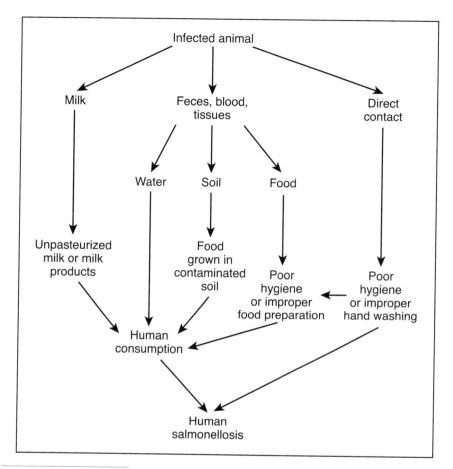

Figure 35. Salmonellosis.

a potential source of infection to people. *Salmonella* can be found in feces, unpasteurized milk, blood, and body tissues.

Livestock can become infected during transport, at fairs, and at auctions, if they come in contact with infected animals. The newly infected livestock will then carry the *Salmonella*, either to their final destination or back home, where they will become a new source of infection to other animals or people.

Pets, especially those with diarrhea, can pass *Salmonella* in their feces. Transmission to people occurs when people do not wash their hands after coming in contact with the feces.

Reptiles, like snakes, iguanas, and turtles, commonly shed *Salmonella*; people need to wash their hands after handling any reptile, even the healthy looking ones.

Person-to-person transmission can occur if infected people do not wash their hands after using the bathroom and then handle food.

Cross-contamination can result when uncontaminated food is placed on a surface previously used for contaminated food.

Flies can transmit *Salmonella* on their feet as they travel from contaminated food to uncontaminated food.

SALMONELLOSIS IN ANIMALS

Salmonellosis in animals may or may not be apparent. Some animals are carriers that shed *Salmonella* at various intervals. Shedding may be brief, or it may occur over a long time. Other animals may develop a latent infection, in which the *Salmonella* organisms enter the blood system and travel to lymph nodes, where they lie dormant. Stress will most commonly cause the dormant organisms to become active.

Because salmonellosis is a disease of the gastrointestinal tract, diarrhea, sometimes bloody, is the most common clinical sign observed.

RUMINANTS

Salmonellosis affects calves primarily and is stress-related, with a high mortality rate. Adult cattle also can be affected. The clinical signs start with high fever, followed by severe diarrhea and abdominal pain. Abortion may occur. Carrier animals shed *Salmonella* in feces and milk. Salmonellosis is not common in sheep and goats in the United States.

PIGS

From *Salmonella*, pigs develop necrotic enteritis, which is usually brought on by stress and will lead to bloody diarrhea. In young pigs, the stress of weaning and vaccination, along with an unsanitary environment, can cause salmonellosis. Contaminated pork is a common source of infection for people.

HORSES

Salmonellosis in horses can cause late abortion in mares, arthritis in colts, and enteritis in all horses. Horses are not a common source of infection for people in the United States.

DOGS AND CATS

Dogs and cats can be carrier animals or can become clinically ill with a *Salmonella* infection. Dogs transmit salmonellosis to people more often than cats do.

FOWL

Chickens, turkeys, and ducks are some of the most important sources of human salmonellosis. Raw eggs can also be a source of *Salmonella*. The outside shell can become contaminated with infected feces, and the interior can become infected before the shell is formed. Some foods that may not obviously contain raw eggs are usually the homemade variety of hollandaise sauce, Caesar salad dressing, ice cream, mayonnaise, cookie dough, eggnog, and frostings.

SALMONELLOSIS IN HUMANS

Not everyone exposed to *Salmonella* will become ill. When illness does occur, it will manifest itself as diarrhea, possibly bloody, abdominal cramps, and fever between 12 and 72 hours after infection. Other clinical signs may include headache, vomiting, and muscle aches. Without treatment most people will recover within a week. It may take some people months before their bowel movements are completely back to normal.

In some cases, the organism may pass into the blood stream and be distributed throughout the body, causing organ damage and possibly death.

A few people who seemingly recover from salmonellosis will develop Reiter syndrome, which affects the joints, eyes, and urogenital tract. The syndrome can last for months or years and usually affects the knees, ankles, and feet, causing pain and swelling at the point where the tendons attach to the bones. It can also affect the lower-back joints. The conjunctivae of the eyes will become inflamed, as will the organs of the urogenital system, in both men and women. *Salmonella* is not the only organism that may result in Reiter syndrome. *Chlamydia* is the most common cause, but *Shigella*, *Yersinia*, and *Campylobacter* may also give rise to Reiter syndrome.

DIAGNOSIS

In people, salmonellosis is diagnosed through laboratory tests that include culturing the feces of sick people. Serologic testing is also used. Once salmonellosis has been diagnosed, further testing to identify which serotype is involved will help determine which antibiotic can be used, if treatment becomes necessary.

In animals, diagnosis is based on fecal culture and serologic testing.

TREATMENT

Treatment for salmonellosis is usually not needed; most people and animals will recover without any medical intervention. Rehydration is essential for those with diarrhea. People should not take antidiarrheal medication, because that can prolong the disease. Antibiotics may become necessary in severe cases. Extremely ill people and animals may have to be hospitalized.

PREVENTION

There is no vaccine to protect against salmonellosis. Because *Salmonella* bacteria are so widespread, it is virtually impossible to make all food free from contamination. The best prevention is to limit possible exposure. This is best accomplished by observing the basic rules of food safety:

- Wash hands thoroughly with warm water and soap after using the bathroom, changing a diaper, or contact with animals; always wash hands before handling food.
- Wash hands thoroughly after handling pets or their feces. Make sure children also wash their hands.
- Do not keep reptiles as pets, especially if there are young children, elderly people, or people with compromised immune systems present. If reptiles are present, wash hands thoroughly after handling them.
- Consider all meat, poultry, vegetables, and milk or milk products contaminated, and handle them accordingly.
- Buy only pasteurized milk and milk products, and inspected meat and eggs. Do not eat foods containing raw or undercooked eggs.
- Wash and properly store all vegetables and fruits.
- Wrap meats in plastic bags to prevent the juices from dripping on other food.
- Refrigerate foods promptly.
- Thaw frozen foods in the refrigerator.
- Avoid cross-contamination from contaminated food to uncontaminated food.
- Avoid eating raw or undercooked meats and poultry. Cook poultry to an internal temperature of 170° to 180° F; use a meat thermometer to be certain foods are properly cooked.
- People with diarrhea should not prepare or serve food to others.
- People with diarrhea should not swim in public pools or lakes.

In animals, prevention is more difficult, and includes the following precautions:

- Carrier animals must be identified and eliminated from a herd or flock.
- Food handling must be controlled to avoid contamination.
- Animal food that contains bone, meat, or fish meal should be avoided, as it can be a source of infection.
- Vaccines are available for a few serotypes but do not offer protection for all the zoonotic serotypes.

NOTE

Since 1976 it has been against the law to sell or distribute turtles with a shell, or *carapace*, less than 4 inches long. The passage of this law followed a fad of buying baby turtles for children as small, easy-to-care-for pets. A turtle, shallow water dish, and plastic palm tree were sold as an inexpensive package by distributors and pet stores. Many people, especially children, developed salmonellosis from these turtles, because the turtles were small and could easily be placed in a child's mouth or because people did not wash their hands after handling the turtles. The mortality rate for the turtles was near 100% because people did not know how to properly care for them, nor did they realize that the turtles would soon outgrow the small bowl and would have to be moved to a larger aquarium. The law has been largely forgotten, and some tourist places are again selling baby turtles or giving them away free when the bowl and food are purchased.

SCABIES

Scabies is a skin disease caused by mites. It is also known as *sarcoptic mange*, *sarcoptic itch*, and the *7-year itch*. Normally an animal species has its own species of mite that causes scabies, and other animal species, including humans, are not affected by that particular species of mite. In other words, it is not a zoonotic problem. However, when people come in repeated or prolonged, close contact with an animal with scabies, temporary *pseudo-scabies* may develop.

MORBIDITY: +
MORTALITY: +
ETIOLOGY: PARASITIC

Scabies is caused by *Sarcoptes scabiei*. Animals and people are infested by their own subspecies of *S. scabiei*, which prefer to live on a specific type of host animal. Human scabies is caused by *S. scabiei* var. *hominis*. Some of the other sarcoptic mites that can be found on other animals, and temporarily on people, are *S. scabiei* var. *canis* (dogs), *S. scabiei* var. *bovis* (cattle), *S. scabiei* var. *equi* (horses), *S. scabiei* var. caprae (goats), and *S. scabiei* var. *suis* (pigs).

A different mite, *Notoedres cati*, causes a disease similar to scabies in cats. This mite may also temporarily infest humans or other animals.

S. scabiei females make tiny burrows into the skin in which to lay their eggs. After about 3 weeks the eggs hatch, and the immature mites come to the opening of the burrow, mature, mate, and move on to make other burrows (Figure 36). The presence of the mites, mite eggs, and mite waste materials causes an allergic reaction in the host, which results in intense itching. Tiny red blisters or bumps develop on the skin, which is also inflamed.

It is while the adult mites are on the skin, rather than in the burrows, that they can be transferred to other animals or people. From a zoonotic standpoint, it is also at this time that the mites may be transferred to an atypical host, such as a person. The mites make their burrows, and the atypical host has an allergic reaction, but the mites die in a couple of days, and the itching goes away.

N. cati has a similar life cycle, but it is the immature mites that are transferred to other animals or people.

HOSTS

S. scabiei is found on warm-blooded animals. The mites tend to be host specific, with little transmission to other animal species or people.

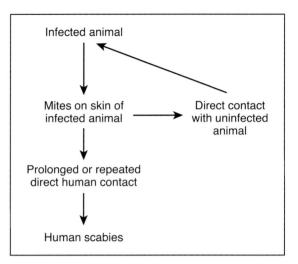

FIGURE 36. Scabies.

TRANSMISSION

Scabies is transmitted from an animal or person with an *S. scabiei* infestation to another animal or person by direct contact. Casual contact, such as shaking hands, does not transmit scabies. Most transmission occurs among animals of like species. Occasionally, people who have repeated, close, prolonged contact with an infested animal may be infested by mites from that animal. Dogs are a common source of this type of transmission.

SCABIES IN ANIMALS

Scabies caused by *S. scabiei* is a disease characterized by intense, persistent itching. With dogs being the one exception, lesions start in areas that have little or no hair in all other common domestic animals, usually around the face, neck, ears, and shoulders. In dogs, the lesions start on the ventral abdomen, chest, ears, and legs (Figure 37).

Scabies in cats caused by *N. cati* looks the same as sarcoptic mange in other animals.

SCABIES IN HUMANS

Scabies occurs in all people, regardless of their social status, hygiene, or environment. Because *S. scabiei* is transmitted by direct contact, scabies is seen more often in crowded situations, like hospitals and nursing homes. Like most diseases, it most often affects the elderly, young children, and people with compromised immune systems.

S. scabiei prefers warm, protected places, so they make their burrows in areas between the fingers, at the belt line, under the nails, in skin folds, and in the groin area (Figures 38 and 39). They also like the skin under bracelets, rings, and watches. Adult female mites are just barely visible without any magnification. They are about the size of the period at the end of this sentence. The burrows are also very small and measure about 2 to 3 mm long.

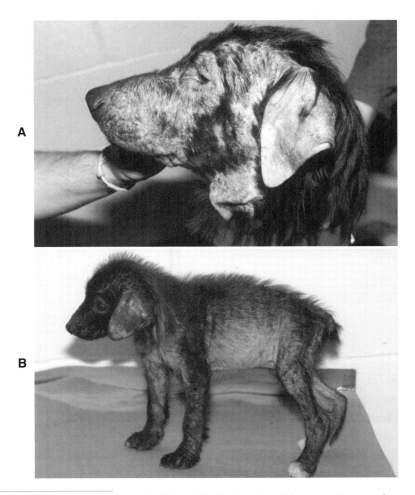

FIGURE 37.   Scabies in dogs. **A,** Generalized alopecia with a crusting popular dermatitis affecting the head and neck of a young adult dog. **B,** Generalized alopecia and crusts affecting a puppy.

Continued

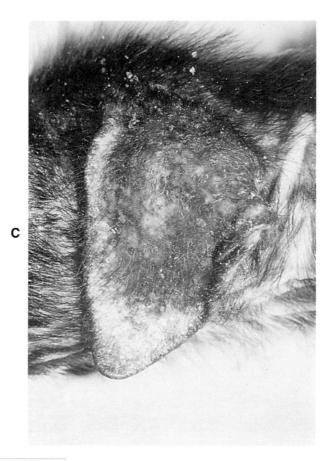

C

FIGURE 37, cont'd.   **C,** Alopecic ear margins, characteristic of scabies. (From Medleau L, Hnilica KA: *Small animal dermatology: a color atlas and therapeutic guide,* ed 2, St Louis, 2006, Saunders.)

A relentless, intense itching gradually develops over a matter of weeks, as more mite eggs are hatched and young mites emerge from the burrows. The itching reportedly worsens at night, but that may be because there is not as much to distract the person from the itch at that time. Tiny, red bumps that look like hives appear, an allergic reaction to the mites, mite eggs, and mite waste material.

DIAGNOSIS

Diagnosis of scabies, in all animals and people, is based on the clinical signs, especially the intense itching. The physician or veterinarian may just need a

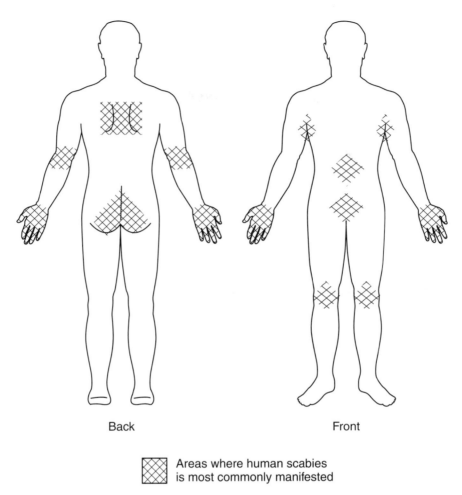

Back   Front

Areas where human scabies
is most commonly manifested

FIGURE 38.   Areas where scabies is most commonly manifested.

magnifying glass to see the mites on the skin. A skin scraping of the affected area may produce mites, but because so few mites can cause the clinical signs, it's easy to miss them. Repeated skin scrapings might be necessary to find mites.

TREATMENT

There are treatments available for both people and animals with scabies. In many cases everyone who has close, prolonged contact with the infested person, especially a sexual partner, is treated also. It is not necessary to get

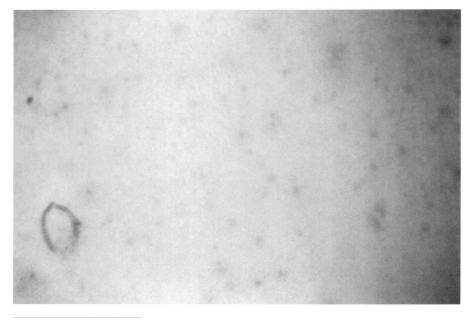

FIGURE 39.   Scabies in a human. (Courtesy Public Health Image Library, PHIL 3972, Centers for Disease Control and Prevention, Atlanta, 1975.)

an exterminator to get rid of mites in a house, kennel, stable, or barn because the mites do not survive off-host for very long. All bedding and linens must be washed.

If the treatment is effective, the mites will be dead within 24 to 48 hours, and the person or animal will no longer be contagious. The itching, however, may take weeks longer to resolve.

PREVENTION

For people, the best way to prevent being infested with *S. scabiei* from animals is to have any animal that develops an intense, persistent itch checked by a veterinarian. If scabies is diagnosed, the animal must be treated. During the treatment avoid prolonged, close contact with the infested animal.

STAPHYLOCOCCOSIS

Staphylococcus aureus causes a variety of diseases. In people it is the cause of skin infections, eye infections, toxic-shock syndrome, and food poisoning. In fact, it is responsible for one of the most common forms of food poisoning in people. In animals it has been associated with skin infections and abscesses in a variety of species; tonsillitis in dogs; septicemia in poultry; and mastitis in cattle, ewes, nanny goats, and sows. We will focus on human staphylococcal food poisoning and the role animals play in its development.

MORBIDITY: ++
MORTALITY: +
ETIOLOGY: BACTERIAL

S. aureus is a gram-positive bacterium that is found on the skin, in the nose, and in the throat in about one third of the human population, as well as in a wide variety of mammals and birds. It can also be found on surfaces, such as food preparation and serving areas, cooking utensils, and milking machines. Sewage and water can also be contaminated. *S. aureus* can live in high salt and sugar concentrations where other bacteria would not survive. It grows best between 68° and 99° F.

Some strains of *S. aureus* produce toxins that are ultimately responsible for clinical signs associated with food poisoning. If the food is contaminated with one of the toxin-producing strains of *S. aureus*, the organism multiplies, and eventually starts producing one of seven toxins. These toxins are extremely heat-resistant and cannot be inactivated by boiling or pasteurization, even though the bacteria that produced the toxins will be killed.

S. aureus is commonly found in cuts, pimples, and abscesses in both people and animals.

HOSTS

S. aureus is found in and on people and many other mammals and birds. Most people who carry *S. aureus* appear healthy.

TRANSMISSION

Humans are the primary source of *S. aureus* in food poisoning that arises from contamination by *S. aureus* toxins. The most common mode of transmission occurs when food is prepared by someone with a skin infection or when food is stored at room temperature. The most susceptible foods are those prepared by hand, which require a lot of handling such as chopping or mixing, and that are not cooked. Bacteria can live and produce toxins in these foods. Common foods in this category are puddings, cream-filled pastries, custards, salads (especially if they contain mayonnaise), sandwich fillings, egg products, milk, dairy products, cream pies, cold meats, and baked goods. There is an increase in the incidence of staphylococcal food poisoning during warm months, because food is often served outdoors and not kept at the proper temperature.

Transmission can also occur when unpasteurized milk or cheeses made from unpasteurized milk are ingested. Even if the milk is pasteurized, *S. aureus* toxins present in the milk before it was pasteurized will survive the pasteurization process. Cooking/pasteurization make foods safer by reducing the numbers of living bacteria that can produce toxins. Once produced, the toxins can withstand temperatures higher than the bacteria that produced them. Ham is one of the most common sources of infection because the *S. aureus* survives the salty curing process. Sneezing on food can also cause *S. aureus* contamination.

STAPHYLOCOCCAL INFECTIONS IN ANIMALS

Animals do not appear susceptible to *S. aureus* food poisoning. *S. aureus* infections are commonly associated with skin diseases, mastitis, septicemia, and abscess formation in many species of animals. Unpasteurized milk and the cheeses made from the unpasteurized milk of cows, ewes, and nanny goats has been the source of the toxin in a number of human infections. In these cases, the *S. aureus* was transmitted to people either through handling the animals or eating contaminated dairy products.

STAPHYLOCOCCAL FOOD POISONING IN HUMANS

Staphylococcal food poisoning in people has an extremely short incubation period; although some will get ill within 30 minutes, the usual range is from 1 to 6 hours. The time of onset of symptoms depends on the person's susceptibility to the *S. aureus* toxin, how much food was eaten, and how much toxin was in the food.

Clinical signs include nausea, vomiting, abdominal cramping, and diarrhea, with a mild fever, or no fever at all. The vomiting can last up to 24 hours.

DIAGNOSIS

Diagnosis of staphylococcal food poisoning is based on history and physical signs. Often one food dish will make many people acutely ill. Fecal samples can be cultured for *S. aureus*, if necessary.

TREATMENT

Most people will recover within 2 to 3 days, without medical intervention. In most cases people just need to keep themselves hydrated during recovery. Some people will become so dehydrated from vomiting and diarrhea that they will have to be hospitalized to restore hydration. Antibiotics are not indicated in the treatment of staphylococcal food poisoning because it is caused by the presence of *S. aureus* toxins, not the actual bacteria. The antibiotics would have no effect on the toxins.

PREVENTION

There is no vaccine to protect against staphylococcal food poisoning. Because staphylococci are so widespread, it is imperative that people preparing and serving food take precautions to keep food safe. This is best accomplished by observing the basic rules of food safety, as follows:

- Wash hands thoroughly with warm water and soap before and after handling food and after using the bathroom or changing diapers.
- When buying refrigerated foods, get them home and properly store them as soon as possible. Food should be cooked, refrigerated, or frozen within 2 hours. Wrap meats in plastic bags to keep meat juices from dripping onto other foods. Keep refrigerator temperature set at, or under, 40° F.
- Buy only pasteurized milk and dairy products.
- Cool leftovers in the refrigerator, partially covered. Cover completely once they are thoroughly cooled.
- Cook foods to recommended temperatures. Leftovers should be heated to at least 165° F.
- Be aware that it is risky to eat raw or undercooked foods, especially pork, beef, fish, clams, and oysters.
- When serving food, keep hot foods at 165° F or above and cold foods at 40° F or colder.
- Follow package information on how to use and store food. Pay attention to expiration dates. Contaminated food does not always smell or look bad, so "when in doubt, throw it out."

TAPEWORMS (CESTODES)

Tapeworms are flat worms that live in the intestinal tracts of their hosts. Adult tapeworms cause little damage to their hosts beyond robbing the host of some micronutrients, such as vitamins. Adult tapeworms are visible to the naked eye and range in size from 0.04 inches to 50 feet long. An infection of tapeworms is called *cestodiasis*.

MORBIDITY: +
MORTALITY: +
ETIOLOGY: PARASITIC

Adult tapeworms are found in the intestinal tracts of their *definitive*, or *final*, hosts. Each adult tapeworm consists of a head (scolex), which attaches the tapeworm to the intestinal wall, neck, and various numbers of segments, developing from the neck region. As new segments are formed at the neck, older segments are pushed back. Tapeworms are hermaphroditic; each segment has two sets of male and female reproductive organs, which will fill the segment with fertile eggs as the segment is pushed back from the neck. When the segment is full of eggs, it detaches itself from the adult tapeworm and is passed in the feces (Figure 40).

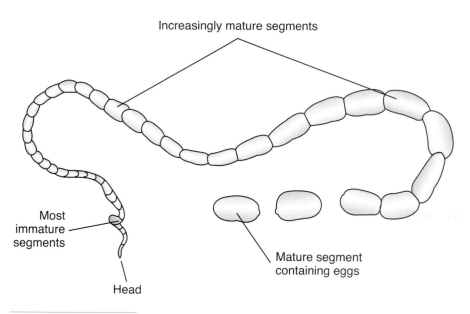

FIGURE 40. Tapeworm morphology.

Each genus and species of tapeworm has at least one *intermediate* host, which ingests the tapeworm eggs. After the eggs hatch, the immature tapeworms migrate out of the intestine of the intermediate host and travel to various tissues in the body, depending on the genus of tapeworm. The immature tapeworm enters tissue in the intermediate host and is enclosed in a cyst, in which young tapeworms develop to an infective stage. *Definitive* hosts are infected by eating the cystic tissues of *intermediate* hosts infected with immature tapeworms.

There are three tapeworms of zoonotic importance in North America: *Dipylidium caninum, Diphyllobothrium latum,* and *Echinococcus spp.*

DIPYLIDIUM CANINUM

Dipylidium caninum is also known as *common dog tapeworm, flea tapeworm, cucumber seed tapeworm,* and *creeping seeds.*

HOSTS

The definitive hosts for *D. caninum* are dogs, cats, foxes, and sometimes humans. The intermediate host is a flea or a louse.

TRANSMISSION

Adult tapeworm segments are passed in the host's feces (Figure 41). These segments look like cucumber seeds or grains of rice and are sometimes seen around the anus of the host or in the feces. After the segments are passed, they can move around. They eventually dry up and release egg packets. The egg packets are then eaten by flea or louse larvae, and hatch in the larvae's small intestines. The larval form of the *tapeworm* then penetrates the intestinal wall of its tiny host and forms cysts in the body cavity. As the flea or louse matures, the tapeworm larva matures, to an infective, cystic stage. The final host is infected by eating a flea or louse infected with immature tapeworms (Figure 42).

DISEASE IN ANIMALS

Dogs, cats, and foxes are usually not much affected by the presence of tapeworms. Dogs may "scoot" or drag their hindquarters to relieve irritation when there are segments stuck to the anal region.

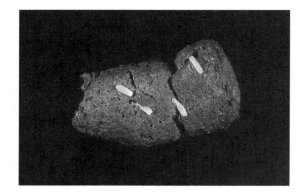

FIGURE 41. Tapeworm segments in dog feces. (From Hendrix CM, Robinson E: *Diagnostic parasitology for veterinary technicians,* ed 3, St Louis, 2006, Mosby.)

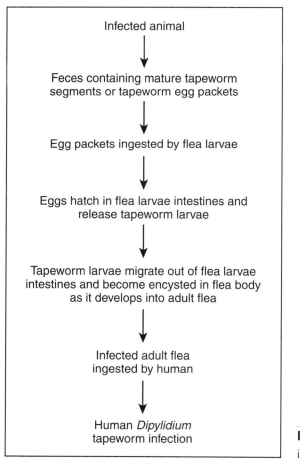

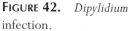

FIGURE 42. *Dipylidium* infection.

Disease in Humans

D. caninum infection is seen most often in children. The only way a person can become infected with D. caninum is to eat a flea or louse larva. Most people with D. caninum infection do not exhibit any clinical signs. Some may develop diarrhea, abdominal pain, and perianal itching from the presence of segments.

Diagnosis

Diagnosis of D. caninum infection is based on finding tapeworm segments that look like cucumber seeds or grains of rice under an animal's tail, around the anus, or on feces passed by the animal. Because the eggs are released in packets, they might not be found on a routine microscopic fecal examination unless the egg packet has broken.

Children infected with D. caninum will pass segments in their stool or have segments, which are irritating and cause itching, stuck to the skin around the anus.

Treatment

Drugs are available to kill adult tapeworms in both animals and humans. After tapeworms have been killed, they are usually digested by the host, so there may be no adult tapeworms passed in the feces.

Prevention

The best prevention is parasite control. Without fleas and lice, there can be no D. caninum. If tapeworms are detected in pets, have them treated. Clean up after pets, especially if they defecate in public areas such as parks or near sidewalks. Do not let children play around areas soiled with dog or cat feces. Make sure children wash their hands after playing with dogs and cats or when they come in from playing outdoors.

It is important to note that sometimes the presence of D. caninum is the first indication that fleas are present in a household.

DIPHYLLOBOTHRIUM LATUM

Diphyllobothrium latum is also known as the broad fish tapeworm. At one time infection with D. latum was known as Jewish or Scandinavian housewife's disease because these women were known to taste gefilte fish, or fish balls, before they were fully cooked. This is rarely seen today. Recent cases of *D. latum* infestation have been associated with eating sushi and sashimi, and in particular, salmon. *D. latum* is a large tapeworm that can reach lengths of up to 32 feet in humans.

HOSTS

The definitive hosts for adult *D. latum* tapeworms are fish-eating mammals, such as bears, cats, dogs, wolves, raccoons, otters, and humans. The intermediate hosts are tiny aquatic crustaceans and fresh water fish, such as minnows, trout, perch, walleyed pike, and salmon. Humans are infected only if they eat raw, infected fish.

TRANSMISSION

The host passes infected feces into bodies of fresh water. The eggs hatch, and the first immature stage of the tapeworm is ingested by tiny aquatic crustaceans. These immature tapeworms migrate to the body cavities of the crustaceans, which become food for small freshwater fish, such as minnows. The minnows' flesh becomes infected with immature tapeworms, and a final host could become infected at this point if it ate raw minnows. When minnows are eaten by larger fish, the flesh of those fish becomes infected. The final host becomes infected from eating the infected fish, either raw or undercooked. Immature tapeworms mature in the intestines of the final host and pass eggs in the host's feces (Figure 43).

DISEASE IN ANIMALS

In pets, infection with *D. latum* is usually not apparent because eggs, rather than grossly visible segments, are passed. Eggs are released individually from segments that do not break off from the adult tapeworm. Intermittently, several segments that have discharged their eggs may break off from the adult tapeworm and be passed in the feces. These are grossly visible but may be missed by the owner.

DISEASE IN HUMANS

D. latum is the largest parasite found in humans in North America. Infection with *D. latum* is usually not associated with any clinical signs. Rarely, an infected

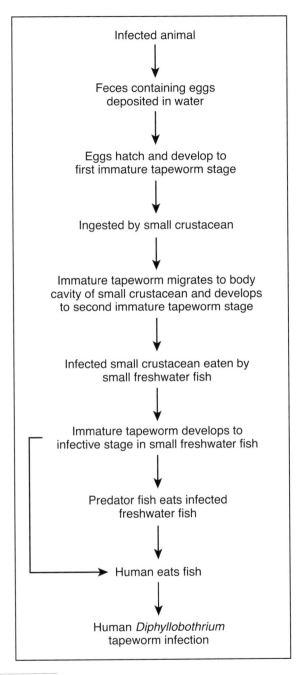

FIGURE 43. *Diphyllobothrium* infection.

person may complain of diarrhea, abdominal pain, vomiting, fatigue, dizziness, and numbness in fingers and toes. Intestinal obstruction is possible when many large tapeworms are present. The adult tapeworm utilizes the host's vitamin B_{12}, which can lead to a deficiency. Vitamin B_{12} is necessary for red blood cell formation, and a deficiency can lead to anemia.

DIAGNOSIS

Diagnosis of *D. latum* infection is based on finding eggs in a microscopic fecal examination. Occasionally strips of segments also may be found in feces.

TREATMENT

Drugs are available for animals and humans that will kill adult tapeworms.

PREVENTION

Cook all fish thoroughly. Freezing fish for at least 24 hours or pickling the fish will kill the infective larvae. Smoking the fish may not kill all the larvae.

ECHINOCOCCUS GRANULOSUS AND MULTIOCULARIS

Echinococcus spp. are the most important zoonotic tapeworms in humans. Echinococcosis in humans is called *hydatid disease* or *cystic hydatid disease* if it is caused by *E. granulosus* and *alveolar hydatid disease* if it is caused by *E. multiocularis*. Hydatid disease is seen in sheep-raising areas of the United States, especially in Utah, California, Arizona, and New Mexico. Alveolar hydatid disease is seen in the north central United States, from Montana to Ohio, and in Alaska and Canada.

HOSTS

Dogs and other canines are the definitive hosts for *E. granulosus*. Many warm-blooded vertebrates, including cattle, sheep, and goats, are the intermediate hosts. Dogs, wild foxes, coyotes, and cats are the definitive hosts for *E. multiocularis*. Rodents, such as voles, shrews, and lemmings, are the intermediate hosts.

Transmission

Echinococcus spp. life cycles are typical of other tapeworm life cycles (Figure 44). The tapeworm eggs are passed in the feces of the final host and are ingested by the intermediate host. *E. granulosus* eggs are passed in canine feces and ingested by an intermediate host. Dogs are reinfected when they eat the infected tissues of cattle, sheep, or goats. Humans are considered dead-end hosts for *E. granulosus*.

Humans and rodents become intermediate hosts infected with *E. multiocularis* by eating anything contaminated with the definitive host's feces. Infection can come from ingesting food contaminated with feces from dogs, coyotes, or foxes, which can happen with herbs, berries, or greens gathered from the wild. People can be infected by petting a cat or dog that has come in contact with feces from infected hosts. The eggs passed in the feces are very small and stick to anything they come in contact with. If a dog did a "scent roll"

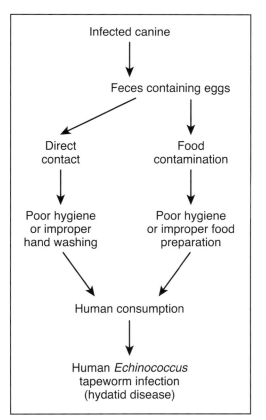

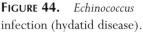

Figure 44.   *Echinococcus* infection (hydatid disease).

in infected feces, the eggs could stick to the dog's coat and be transferred to anyone who pets it. People could become infected by not washing their hands after petting the animal and then transferring the eggs to their mouths.

DISEASE IN ANIMALS

The adult *Echinococcus* tapeworm is small (3 to 5 mm), so it causes little damage in the definitive host. Once the eggs are ingested by the intermediate host, they hatch in the intestines. The larvae penetrate the intestinal walls and migrate to specific tissues in the intermediate host. *E. granulosus* larvae migrate primarily to the liver, where they become enclosed in a cyst called a *hydatid cyst*. The larvae also migrate to the lungs, spleen, and other organs, where they also form hydatid cysts. *E. multiocularis* larvae migrate to the liver, lungs, brain, and other organs, where they form hydatid cysts. Each hydatid cyst contains many infective, immature tapeworms, which will become many adult tapeworms in the definitive host when the cysts are ingested. The damage done by the hydatid cyst in the intermediate host depends on the size of the cyst and the tissue in which it is located. Many animal intermediate hosts are not affected by the hydatid cysts.

DISEASE IN HUMANS

The damage done by hydatid cysts in body tissues depends on the size of the cyst and the tissue in which it is located. Alveolar hydatid disease (AHD), caused by *E. multiocularis*, is caused by hydatid cysts primarily in the liver (Figure 45) but also in other tissues, including the brain. Because of the potential brain involvement, infection with *E. multiocularis* is more likely to be fatal to humans than *E. granulosus*. The hydatid cysts are slow-growing, so clinical signs may not become evident until many years following initial infection.

DIAGNOSIS

Echinococcosis is diagnosed by finding eggs in the feces of the definitive host. In the intermediate host, there are blood tests that detect antibodies against *Echinococcus spp*. Aspiration of a hydatid cyst will reveal the presence of the immature tapeworms. CAT scans and MRI scans are also used to detect the presence of hydatid cysts.

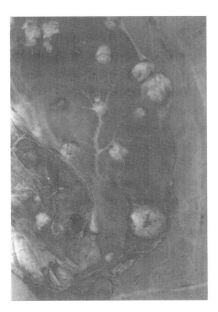

FIGURE 45.   Hydatid cysts in the liver. (From Knottenbelt DC, Pascoe RR: *Color atlas of diseases and disorders of the horse,* London, 1994, Mosby.)

TREATMENT

There are drugs available to control adult tapeworms in definitive hosts. In humans, the treatment of choice for hydatid cysts is surgery. There are newer drugs available that can be used in conjunction with the surgery or alone if surgery is not an option.

PREVENTION

Echinococcosis can be controlled by preventing dogs and cats from eating intermediate hosts. Animals should not be fed uncooked meat or viscera. Also, rodent populations should be controlled. People who are at higher risk for becoming infected with *Echinococcus spp.* are hunters, trappers, veterinarians, veterinary technicians, and others who might have contact with wild animals or their feces. Prevention includes the following precautions:

- Wear gloves when handling foxes, coyotes, or wild canines, whether they are dead or alive. Hunters should wear gloves when cleaning animals.
- Wild animals should not be kept as pets, nor should they be encouraged to hang around a home.
- Cats and dogs should not be allowed to wander freely, where they can eat rodents.

- People should wash their hands after handling pets.
- Fence in gardens to keep out wild animals that might defecate on growing plants.
- Wash all wild-picked food before eating it. Do not eat food directly from the ground.

INTERESTING NOTE

The "Hollywood Tapeworm Diet" was supposedly used by actors and models as a means of losing weight. It was thought that if a person was intentionally infected with tapeworms, the tapeworms would deprive the person of nutrients and cause the person to become thinner. This is not likely to happen because a tapeworm will normally absorb micronutrients that are usually not needed by the person. This is an interesting if not somewhat bizarre diet that has been classified as a true urban legend.

TOXOPLASMOSIS

Cats have gotten a bad rap about how they transmit toxoplasmosis to humans and how they cause spontaneous abortion in women and blindness and mental retardation in newborns and older children. While it is true that cats are the only definitive host for the infective stage of the *Toxoplasma* organism, they are *not* the most common source of human infection. The most efficient way to get toxoplasmosis from a cat is to eat the cat undercooked!

MORBIDITY: +++
MORTALITY: +
ETIOLOGY: PARASITIC

Toxoplasmosis is caused by *Toxoplasma gondii*, a microscopic, intracellular pro-tozoan. Its life cycle has a sexual phase and an asexual phase. The sexual phase takes place only in the walls of the small intestines of wild and domestic cats, resulting in oocysts that are passed in the cats' feces. A cat will shed millions of oocysts per day, for about 2 to 3 weeks, and is then done shedding oocysts—for life.

The asexual phase occurs when the oocysts become infective, or *sporulate*, 1 to 5 days after they are passed in the feces. These oocysts are resistant to environmental conditions and can remain infective for over a year. When the sporulated oocysts are ingested by an animal, they go to the animal's small intestine, enter the *tachyzoite stage*, penetrate the intestinal wall, and travel to other parts of the body in lymph and blood. During this stage, tachyzoites rapidly multiply in the cytoplasms of monocytes and macrophages. The tachy-zoite (asexual) stage, which is called the *active* or *acute phase*, lasts until the host's immune system produces some immunity—about 2 weeks. Once the immunity develops, the tachyzoites slow their multiplication rate and become bradyzoites, which accumulate in the cytoplasm of tissue cells and form cysts. The cysts can be found anywhere in the body, but are most commonly seen in skeletal muscle, myocardium, and brain tissue. The *bradyzoite (asexual) stage* is the *inactive phase*. Cysts can remain in the host for the rest of its life. If the host's immunity is somehow suppressed, the bradyzoites can become rapidly multiplying tachyzoites again, resulting in a latent or chronic infection (Figure 46).

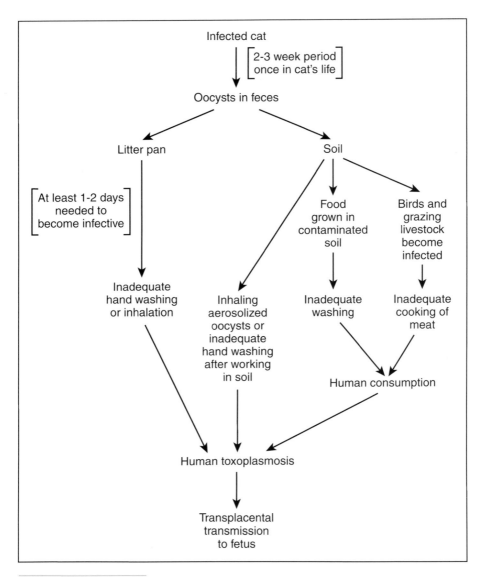

FIGURE 46. Toxoplasmosis.

HOSTS

Cats are the only definitive host for *T. gondii*. This means cats are the only animals that harbor the organism during the organism's sexual, adult phase. Other animals, including people, that become infected with *T. gondii* are considered intermediate hosts. Most species of warm-blooded animals and birds are susceptible to *T. gondii* infection.

TRANSMISSION

Transmission from cats to animals occurs when animals come in contact with sporulated *Toxoplasma* oocysts. The oocysts can be found where cats defecate, such as moist soil, litter boxes, sand boxes, flower beds, and gardens. Rodents, birds, and other small animals can become infected and infect the cats that prey on them. This perpetuates the life cycle in cats. Cats also can become infected by coming in direct contact with the feces from other infected cats.

Animals on pasture, such as sheep, pigs, goats, and cattle, can ingest the oocysts while they are grazing. Their meat (skeletal muscle) will then become infected with *T. gondii* cysts that can be transmitted to people or other carnivores and scavengers, including cats, that eat the meat raw or undercooked. Undercooked meat, especially lamb, beef, or pork, is the most common source of *T. gondii* infection in people.

Once ingested by any susceptible animal other than a cat, the *Toxoplasma* organisms are released in the intestines, develop to the tachyzoite stage, and go through the migration into body tissues as previously described.

If a cat eats the infected tissues, some of the released *Toxoplasma* organisms stay in the cat's intestines to go through the sexual phase, releasing oocysts in the feces. Other released *Toxoplasma* organisms will develop to the tachyzoite stage, penetrate the intestinal wall, and eventually become bradyzoites encysted in body tissues.

Rarely people can become infected directly from cats if they ingest or breathe in the sporulated oocysts from an infected cat. This can happen when hands become contaminated while changing a litter box or if the litter is dusty enough to allow the oocysts to ride on the dust and be inhaled. Working in soil without gloves and playing in a sandbox are other methods of direct infection from cats. Infection can also occur after eating unwashed vegetables from gardens or after drinking contaminated water. Oocysts can be carried on the wind or in water to distant places.

Transmission can also occur transplacentally in people if a mother is infected near the time she becomes pregnant or soon after. This results in congenital toxoplasmosis, which is the least common but most severe form of toxoplasmosis in people. Congenital toxoplasmosis is also seen in goats and sheep.

Transmission among people can occur through blood transfusions and organ donation.

TOXOPLASMOSIS IN ANIMALS

Many species of animals and birds are susceptible to *T. gondii* infection, but clinical disease is rare.

In sheep and goats, congenital toxoplasmosis can cause abortion and disease in newborn lambs. Adult sheep and goats rarely develop clinical signs.

Dogs are commonly infected but rarely become ill. When clinical disease develops, it resembles canine distemper, which is characterized by fever and respiratory congestion that may develop into bronchitis, pneumonia, and gastroenteritis.

Remember, cats shed oocysts only *once* in their lives, for a period of 2 to 3 weeks. Many cats are infected with *T. gondii* as kittens or young adults. Most of them will be asymptomatic and immune to repeat infections as adults. Clinical toxoplasmosis is characterized primarily by pneumonia of increasing severity. Other signs are nonspecific and include fever, depression, anorexia, and lethargy. Hepatitis may develop. The eyes and central nervous system can be affected, which might be manifested by retinitis, abnormal pupil size, blindness, incoordination, circling, personality change, ear twitching, difficulty chewing and swallowing, and loss of control of urination and defecation.

TOXOPLASMOSIS IN HUMANS

Of the world population, 30% to 50% has been infected with *T. gondii*. In North America, 10% to 20% of the population harbors *T. gondii* cysts. An estimated 60 million people in the United States are currently infected with *T. gondii*, but 80% to 90% of them will never develop clinical signs or will become only mildly ill if they have healthy immune systems. These numbers are important because if the immune system of any of these people becomes suppressed—as in people with HIV/AIDS or people undergoing chemotherapy, on steroids, or taking immunosuppressants after organ transplants—the bradyzoites in tissue cysts may become activated tachyzoites, resulting in latent toxoplasmosis. Every year in the United States, 3000 babies are born with congenital toxoplasmosis.

Unlike congenital toxoplasmosis, toxoplasmosis acquired after birth most often goes undetected or is characterized by mild, flulike or mononucleosis-like symptoms, including swollen lymph nodes in the head and neck, headache, sore throat, and muscle pain that lasts for a few days to a month or more. The incubation period is 1 to 2 weeks. In most cases the disease is self-limiting because it is controlled by the immune system. Severe toxoplasmosis, however, can result in lesions in the eyes and central nervous system.

Latent toxoplasmosis, brought on by immunosuppression, is characterized by central nervous system lesions that result in headache, confusion, seizures, and other neurological signs. If the retina becomes inflamed, blurred vision will result. A fever is usually present, and lymph nodes are enlarged. Respiratory disease and heart disease will commonly develop. In people with HIV/AIDS, repeat infections are common, and the mortality rate is high.

Congenital toxoplasmosis is the most devastating form of the disease in people. Infections that occur in early pregnancy will result in fewer but more severe cases of toxoplasmosis. Infections that occur later in pregnancy will result in more infections but a less severe disease. It is important to note that if a fetus becomes infected, it is asymptomatic at birth most of the time. Most babies infected with congenital toxoplasmosis will show symptoms weeks, months, even years after birth. Even though very few infected babies show signs of toxoplasmosis at birth, some infected babies may already have suffered serious eye or brain damage.

Clinical congenital toxoplasmosis is characterized by central nervous system and ocular disorders. These disorders include mental retardation, hydrocephalus, convulsions, deafness, blindness, or cerebral palsy. Ocular toxoplasmosis is another consequence of congenital toxoplasmosis. It develops as chorioretinitis during a person's 20s and 30s.

DIAGNOSIS

Patient history, clinical signs, and the results of diagnostic tests can lead to a presumptive diagnosis of toxoplasmosis.

There are a number of diagnostic tests available to isolate and observe the parasites in patients. They include lymph node biopsy, examination of respiratory fluid, examination of the retina, and injecting mice with patient blood or other body fluids to see if the mice develop an infection. These tests are complex and are not very reliable.

Serologic testing to determine if the patient has antibodies against *T. gondii* will indicate whether the patient has ever been infected with *T. gondii*. The presence of antibodies can be a good thing, because most animals and people are immune to toxoplasmosis if they've been previously infected. Women who are pregnant or trying to conceive and who have had contact with cats who may have had acute toxoplasmosis may want to have serology testing to see if they have antibodies against *T. gondii*. If they do have the antibodies, it greatly reduces the chances of congenital toxoplasmosis developing in the fetus.

TREATMENT

Most people and animals are not treated for toxoplasmosis because the clinical signs resolve on their own when immunity has developed. There are drugs available if treatment is warranted, such as in people with suppressed immune systems or for women who are pregnant and test negative for *T. gondii* antibodies.

Cats in the acute phase of toxoplasmosis can receive drugs that inhibit *T. gondii* reproduction.

PREVENTION

There are no vaccines currently available for toxoplasmosis.

Women who are pregnant and people who are immunosuppressed do not have to get rid of their cats. However, it may be unwise for these people to adopt kittens or young adult cats, because these are most likely to shed the oocysts.

Steps that can be taken to prevent toxoplasmosis in people include the following:
• Exclude raw and undercooked meat from the diet. Cooking meat to an internal temperature of 158° F (70° C) for at least 15 minutes will kill the cysts. There is some disagreement about whether freezing meat before eating it will kill the cysts. Pickling, salting, or smoking meat will not destroy the cysts.
• Exclude unpasteurized milk and dairy products from the diet. Cysts are sometimes passed in the milk, especially goat milk.
• Do not drink untreated water from streams, lakes, or rivers.
• Wash hands, cutting boards, and utensils in warm, soapy water after handling raw meat.
• Wear gloves when working in potentially infected soil in gardens and flower beds. Wash hands after removing gloves.
• Keep sandboxes tightly covered when children are not playing in them to prevent cats from using them as litter boxes.
• Keep cats healthy by keeping them indoors to prevent them from being exposed to other cats or from eating prey that may be infected.
• Remove feces from litter boxes every day. Remember, it takes oocysts 1 to 5 days to sporulate after being passed in cat feces.

- Do not feed cats raw or undercooked meat. Feed only commercial cat food. This will reduce the possibility of cats becoming infected.
- Some people may prefer to wear gloves when cleaning the litter box. Even so, wash the hands after removing the gloves.
- Pregnant women may feel more comfortable having someone else clean the litter box, even though the chances of becoming infected in this way are slim.

TRICHINOSIS

Trichinosis, also known as *trichinellosis*, is a food-borne disease caused by a small parasite living in muscle tissue and eaten in raw or undercooked meat. The disease has traditionally been associated with eating undercooked pork, but strict federal regulations and education have greatly reduced the incidence of pork-related trichinosis in North America.

MORBIDITY: +
MORTALITY: +
ETIOLOGY: PARASITIC

Trichinosis is caused by the parasitic roundworm *Trichinella spp*. In North America the three most common species involved are *T. spiralis* (found in pigs and rats), *T. murrelli* (found in wild game in temperate regions), and *T. nativa* (found in cold climate–adapted animals such as fox, wolf, walrus, and bear).

Adult *Trichinella* worms mate in the small intestine of a host. Instead of hatching from eggs, the young parasite develops in the adult female parasite until it reaches the larval stage; these larvae are then passed by the adult female. The male dies after mating; the female dies after passing larvae. Both are then passed in the feces. The larvae penetrate the intestinal wall, enter the lymph and blood systems, and are carried to various tissues throughout the body, including the striated muscles (meat). In the muscles larvae curl up, and an individual cyst is formed around each larva. In the cysts the larvae lie dormant until they are liberated by gastric juices when the meat is eaten by another host. Once the larvae are freed from their cysts by the digestion process, they are carried to the small intestine of the new host, where they mature to adults, mate, produce more larvae, and die.

If the meat containing encysted larvae is never eaten, the larvae will eventually die, and the cysts will become calcified. This is what happens in people and in animals that are not on the menu for human or animal consumption. Encysted larvae in pigs have been known to live 11 years.

HOSTS

Carnivores and omnivores are most susceptible to developing trichinosis because they are most apt to eat infected meat. Herbivores, such as horses, can become infected if they eat feed that contains scraps of uncooked, infected meat. Some animals that can be sources of infection are pigs, wolves, ground squirrels, bears (grizzly, polar, and black), walruses, seals, whales, dogs, cats (wild and domestic), rats, foxes, and horses. In the past pigs were the primary sources of infection, because their diet consisted of uncooked garbage containing raw, infected meat. Today, packing plants are federally inspected, and it is against the law to feed raw garbage to pigs intended for market. Homegrown pigs fed raw garbage and never passing through a federally inspected packing plant can still be a source of infection.

TRANSMISSION

Most cases of trichinosis involve eating meat. Transmission occurs when an animal or a person eats raw or undercooked meat from an infected animal. The dormant larvae that were encysted in the muscle tissue (meat) are released from their cysts by stomach juices when they are ingested. From there they complete their life cycles and infect the muscles of the new animal or human host (Figure 47). In North America, people are usually dead-end hosts, as are some animals, such as dogs and horses, as they are not eaten on a regular basis.

Not thoroughly cleaning a meat grinder after grinding infected meat may result in subsequently ground meat becoming infected. If not properly cleaned, other equipment also can harbor infected meat scraps and act as a source of infection.

Transmission from person to person or from person to animal does not occur.

TRICHINOSIS IN ANIMALS

Animals with trichinosis look healthy and do not usually become clinically ill. This is especially significant in wild animals killed for their meat. Every wild animal should be considered potentially infected.

TRICHINOSIS IN HUMANS

Most people who become infected with *Trichinella* will never become clinically ill or will exhibit only mild signs that are often mistaken for the flu. The disease is more common in rural, areas where pigs are raised for personal, not commercial, use.

Trichinosis in humans occurs in two stages. When the adult worms are in the intestines mating and producing larvae that invade the intestinal walls, people will suffer intestinal signs such as diarrhea, abdominal pain, fever,

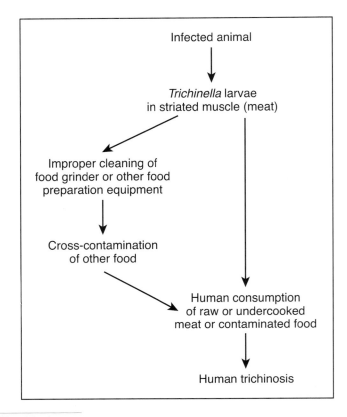

FIGURE 47.   Trichinosis.

vomiting, and lethargy. These signs appear 1 to 2 days after eating infected meat. The severity of the signs depends on how many parasites are present— the more parasites, the more severe the signs.

As the larvae migrate through the body, finding their way to muscles and other body tissues, the second round of symptoms appears, 7 to 11 days later. The larvae seem to prefer certain muscles, which results in some specific signs. For instance, infection in the muscles around the eyes results in swelling of the eyelids; this is considered a hallmark sign of trichinosis. The diaphragm, biceps, and muscles of the jaw, lower back, and neck are other favored muscles. Other signs include bleeding into nail beds, swollen face, bleeding into retinas and sclerae, high fever, chills, cough, joint pain, nonitchy rash, muscle pain and tenderness, weakness, headaches, and sensitivity to light. The symptoms are at their worst about 3 weeks after infection.

Most cases of trichinosis are self-limiting. After the symptoms reach their peak, they gradually begin to subside. This can take several months. The muscle pain and fatigue can last several months beyond the resolution of the other signs.

In severe cases the larvae may cause pneumonia, encephalitis, and heart failure, all of which can be fatal.

Diagnosis

A patient history of eating raw or undercooked meat is the place to start when diagnosing trichinosis. Serologic testing can be used to detect antibodies against the parasite. The migrating larvae cause a sensitivity reaction that results in an increased number of eosinophils in peripheral blood. A blood sample can be examined for this eosinophilia. A muscle biopsy can be examined for the presence of encysted larvae, but the test can be painful and is often unrewarding, especially if the number of cysts is low. Examination of a fecal sample is not a diagnostic test for trichinosis, because the adults and larvae are seldom seen in feces.

Treatment

Drugs are available to treat the parasites *only* when they are in the intestines. Once they encyst in muscles and tissues, the medication cannot reach them. This makes treatment difficult, because the intestinal phase of trichinosis resembles many gastrointestinal diseases. Symptomatic treatment, with painkillers and steroids, is the only treatment option in many cases.

Prevention

The only way to prevent trichinosis in people is to cook all meat thoroughly before eating it:

- Cook meat, including wild game, to an internal temperature of 170° F (77° C), or until the juices run clear.
- Freezing meat less than 6 inches thick at 5° F (−15° C) for 20 days will kill T. spiralis but not necessarily T. nativa, which is found in cold climate–adapted animals. Freezing may not kill all T. murrelli larvae in wild game.
- Cook all meat fed to pigs.
- Do not allow pigs to eat uncooked carcasses of other animals.
- Clean meat grinders and other equipment after each use.
- Smoking, drying, curing, and pickling meat will not kill all of the Trichinella larvae in infected meat.
- Microwaves do not heat meat consistently, so do not rely on them to kill Trichinella larvae.

Trichinosis is still a problem in other countries, so people traveling abroad should be careful about eating raw or undercooked meat, especially pork. It is still common to feed pigs raw garbage in developing countries.

NOTE

Trichinosis has been a reportable disease in the United States since 1966. Cases of human or animal trichinosis must be reported to local, state, and federal health officials.

TULAREMIA

Tularemia is a bacterial infection, commonly known as *rabbit fever* or *deer tick fever*. The disease is endemic to certain areas of the United States and is highly infectious. It has been identified as a possible agent of biological warfare in aerosol form. As few as 10 organisms can cause disease.

MORBIDITY: +
MORTALITY: ++
ETIOLOGY: BACTERIAL

Tularemia is caused by *Francisella tularensis*, a small, gram-negative coccobacillus. The bacterium has a capsule that allows it to survive for several months in water, mud, and decomposing materials, including carcasses.

HOSTS

F. tularensis has been found in over 200 species of vertebrates and invertebrates. The most important hosts in North America are wild rabbits, hares, rodents, pheasants, quail, ticks, and deer flies. Humans are not a natural host. Every state in the United States except Hawaii has reported tularemia. Most cases occur in rural areas in south-central and western states.

TRANSMISSION

Transmission occurs through direct contact with an infected animal, from insect or arthropod bites, or by ingestion of the organism in contaminated food or water. Hunters may come in contact with *F. tularensis* when skinning or dressing infected rabbits or other wild animals.

Ticks have become the most important vector for transmission of tularemia to humans and domestic animals. They also act as a reservoir to carry *F. tularensis* from one geographic area or group of animals to another. Exposure to infected rabbits is the second most common source of tularemia. Horse flies, biting flies, sucking lice, and mosquitoes are other vectors, but not as important as ticks (Figure 48).

F. tularensis can also be aerosolized by riding on particles of dust or mist and can be inhaled. This happens most often during gardening, landscaping, construction, or any activity that disturbs soil. Another less common mode of

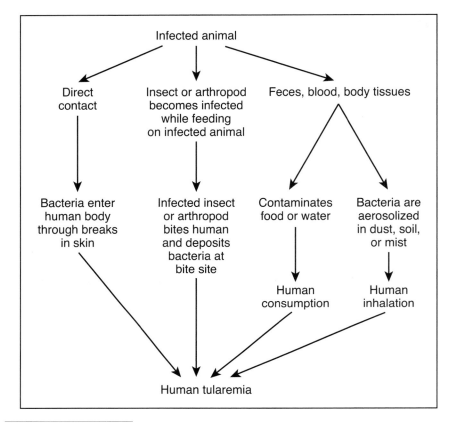

FIGURE 48.   Tularemia.

transmission is handling infected animals or tissues in a laboratory. Person-to-person transmission does not occur.

TULAREMIA IN ANIMALS

Tularemia is more common in wild animals than domestic ones, and is more often fatal in wild animals. Domestic animals are usually considered accidental hosts for *F. tularensis*. Some species are more susceptible than others to developing clinical disease. The incubation period is 1 to 10 days.

WILD RABBITS, HARES, AND RODENTS

Wild rabbits, hares, and rodents are very susceptible to *F. tularensis* infection and are often found dead, having exhibited no observable clinical signs. When clinical signs are present, they include depression, anorexia, incoordination, roughened hair coat, and huddling. Pet rabbits and rodents rarely develop tularemia if they are kept indoors.

SHEEP
Tularemia in sheep can be fatal. It shows up as a seasonal disease that coincides with tick season. The clinical signs include fever, diarrhea, weight loss, dyspnea, polyuria (excessive urination), rigid movements, and isolation from the rest of the flock. Mortality is greatest in lambs, and ewes may abort.

CATS
Cats vary in their susceptibility to *F. tularensis* infection. Some infections are inapparent; others result in septicemia and death. Clinical signs include fever, depression, jaundice, anorexia, weight loss, pneumonia, abscesses, mouth ulcers, splenomegaly (abnormally enlarged spleen), and hepatomegaly (abnormally enlarged liver).

HORSES
Clinical signs of tularemia in horses also coincide with tick season. A heavier tick infestation results in a more severe disease. Affected horses display fever, dyspnea, depression, and incoordination. Tularemia is not common in horses.

DOGS
Dogs are usually not seriously affected by *F. tularensis* infection. When clinical signs appear, they include fever, mucopurulent (part mucus, part pus) discharge from the eyes and nose, pustule formation at the site of a tick bite, enlarged lymph nodes, and anorexia. Dogs probably serve as reservoirs for *F. tularensis* and are maintenance hosts for tick vectors.

CATTLE
Cattle seem to be resistant to clinical disease resulting from *F. tularensis* infection.

TULAREMIA IN HUMANS

Tularemia is a disease primarily of rural areas, where people and animals are more likely to come in contact with ticks and infected animals. A majority of tularemia cases are seen during tick season, and hunters are commonly infected. Veterinarians, veterinary technicians, farmers, foresters, and wildlife specialists who work directly with wildlife are also at increased risk for developing tularemia.

Most people who are exposed to *F. tularensis* become sick in 3 to 5 days, but it can take up to 2 weeks for the clinical signs to appear. There are six types of tularemia, but two of the types are responsible for nearly 100% of tularemia cases. How a person is infected usually determines which form of tularemia will develop.

Ulceroglandular tularemia is by far the most common form. It begins when an ulcer forms at an inoculation site, usually where the person was bitten by an insect or animal (Figure 49). Bacteria then spread from the inoculation site to regional lymph nodes, which become painful and swollen; fever, chills, headache, and lethargy soon develop.

Typhoidal, or *septicemic*, tularemia is the next most common form. Ulcers and enlarged lymph nodes do not develop, but pneumonia does. This makes diagnosis difficult. Also seen are fever, chills, myalgia, lethargy, and weight loss. The mode of transmission is not confirmed, but ingestion is commonly suggested.

The other four forms that are much more uncommon are the *glandular form* (no ulcer forms), *oculoglandular form* (*F. tularensis* enters through the eye),

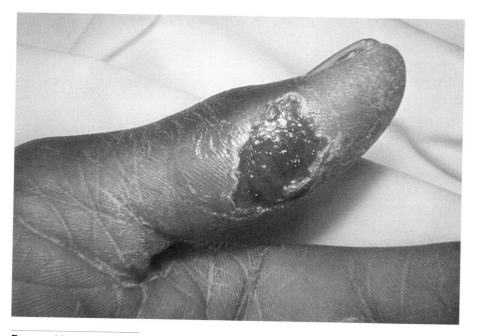

FIGURE 49.   Tularemia in a human, showing ulceration at the site of the bite. (Courtesy Public Health Image Library, PHIL 1344, Centers for Disease Control and Prevention, Atlanta, 1964.)

oropharyngeal form (from ingesting undercooked infected meat, typically rabbit), and the *pneumonic form* (*F. tularensis* is inhaled).

The clinical signs observed correlate to the route of infection. For example, if *F. tularensis* is ingested, mouth sores can develop. People who develop tularemia through inhalation can develop chest pain, dyspnea, bloody sputum, and respiratory failure. Infection through the eye results in a reddened conjunctiva with purulent exudates, corneal ulcers, and enlarged lymph nodes in the head and neck. Complications that have been reported in severe cases of tularemia are meningitis, pericarditis, and osteomyelitis. Of these three, meningitis is the most life-threatening if not treated promptly.

DIAGNOSIS

Serologic tests can detect antibodies against *F. tularensis*. Diagnosis of tularemia in animals is often done at necropsy. Animals or specimens of blood, biopsies, or exudates that are submitted to a diagnostic or reference laboratory must be labeled as potentially tularemia-infected to prevent laboratory personnel from accidentally becoming infected.

People are diagnosed with tularemia by screening for antibodies against *F. tularensis* in their blood. *F. tularensis* can be cultured, but it is difficult to do, and colonies take a long time to grow—up to 3 weeks. Clinical signs, and a history of exposure to ticks or potentially infected rabbits aid in diagnosis.

TREATMENT

Tularemia can be fatal if not treated. Antibiotics and supportive treatment are usually successful, especially if started early.

PREVENTION

There is no vaccine available to prevent tularemia in animals or people. Tick control has become the most important preventive measure in people and animals. Other precautions follow:
• Stay away from areas where ticks are commonly found.
• Use insect repellent containing DEET on exposed skin. Follow the instructions on the repellent container carefully. Wear long pants and long-sleeved shirts. Tuck pants into socks and tuck shirts into pants. Treat clothing with a repellent that contains permethrin. Wear a broad-rimmed hat to protect head and neck.

- Protect pets from tick and fly bites. Flea and tick collars might help.
- Do not let pets or livestock eat parts of diseased animals, especially rabbits.
- People should inspect their own and their animals' entire bodies for ticks.
- Properly remove any ticks found; this means wearing gloves or using a tissue while grasping the tick close to the skin and pulling it out. *Do not use lighted cigarettes, matches, alcohol, or petroleum jelly. Do not squeeze the tick.* Sometimes there is a large, blood-engorged female tick and a smaller, male tick at the same site. Be sure to remove both ticks.
- Properly dispose of ticks by flushing them down the toilet. These ticks don't need to be saved in alcohol for diagnosis.
- Thoroughly clean the area where a tick was removed, and wash hands with warm, soapy water.
- Protect hands with gloves when skinning or dressing rabbits, hares, rodents, pheasants, and quail. Keep hands away from the eyes and wash hands well when finished.
- Clean all instruments and equipment used on potentially infected animals.
- Disinfect surfaces where potentially infected animals have been. Use one part household bleach to nine parts water, and let the solution sit on the surface for 30 minutes.
- Cook rabbit and other wild game thoroughly. Never eat it raw or undercooked.
- Do not drink untreated water, especially in endemic areas where tularemia is more common.
- Consider wearing a face mask and gloves when working in soil, mowing the lawn, clearing weeds, or excavating construction sites.
- Discourage children from touching dead rabbits or other wild animals.

HISTORICAL NOTE

Though the disease had been identified in 1837, it was not given the name *tularemia* until 1911, when a plaguelike disease infected ground squirrels living in Tulare County, California. Dr. Edward Francis subsequently worked with the organism that eventually bore his name.

VIBRIOSIS

Eating raw, undercooked, or improperly refrigerated shellfish can lead to vibriosis, a bacterial disease most commonly seen in areas near the sea. Vibriosis can also occur as a result of wound contamination with seawater.

MORBIDITY: +
MORTALITY: + TO ++++
ETIOLOGY: BACTERIAL

Vibrio parahaemolyticus and *Vibrio vulnificus* are the two organisms responsible for most cases of vibriosis in people. They are curved gram-negative rods that require salt water to survive (halophiles). They are found as natural residents in seawater along the Atlantic coast up to Cape Cod, the Gulf of Mexico coast, and the entire Pacific coast. *Vibrio* grows best during the warmer months of summer when water is warmer.

HOSTS

V. parahaemolyticus and *V. vulnificus* have been isolated from shellfish (including crustaceans, such as lobsters, crabs, and shrimp); mollusks (such as oysters, clams, scallops, cockles, and mussels); fin fish (such as mackerel, tuna, and sardines); seawater; sediment; and plankton.

TRANSMISSION

Oysters are the most common shellfish involved in infection in people. People become infected with *V. parahaemolyticus* and *V. vulnificus* when they eat shellfish that has not been properly stored or cooked. If shellfish are not cleaned and cooled immediately after catching them, the bacteria will multiply rapidly. Even if the shellfish were cooled properly, they can still be infected and must be cooked thoroughly to prevent human infection. The *Vibrio* organisms adhere so tightly to the shellfish intestinal tract that washing the shellfish does not remove them. Freezing does not kill the organisms, and the bacteria can live for several months in frozen seafood.

Person-to-person transmission has not been documented. The presence of *Vibrio spp.* in seawater does not indicate fecal contamination of the water.

Existing wounds can become infected with contaminated seawater, or new wounds can occur by cutting any part of the body with sharp objects, such as fishhooks or coral. The new wounds can also become infected.

VIBRIOSIS IN ANIMALS

V. parahaemolyticus and *V. vulnificus* cause asymptomatic contamination of shell-fish and some fin fish. The presence of *V. parahaemolyticus* and *V. vulnificus* is not apparent because the organisms do not affect the smell, appearance, or taste of the shellfish or fish.

VIBRIOSIS IN HUMANS

Vibriosis that results from eating improperly stored or cooked shellfish is characterized by profuse, watery diarrhea that starts on average 12 to 24 hours after consumption. Fever, nausea, abdominal cramps, chills, and headaches can accompany the diarrhea. The diarrhea is a result of damage to the intestinal wall. The disease is self-limiting in 2 to 3 days or up to a week in immunocompetent people. *V. parahaemolyticus* causes severe gastroenteritis and is more likely to be associated with outbreaks involving numerous people who ate infected shellfish.

V. vulnificus is associated more with individual cases of vibriosis in which the gastroenteritis is not as severe. However, the organism can penetrate the intestinal wall and get into the blood stream, causing septicemia. In immuno-competent people, this can result in skin lesions characterized by erythema, edema, and pain. The lesions do not spread, and necrosis and gangrene are seldom a problem.

In people with certain preexisting conditions, *V. vulnificus* infection can lead to a life-threatening disease, characterized by septic shock, cellulitis, and blistering skin lesions, most often on the legs and arms, and particularly on the palms, fingertips, and soles of the feet (Figure 50). The painful lesions resemble *necrotizing fasciitis* and spread rapidly. Necrosis and gangrene may follow, necessitating amputation to stop the spread of the lesions.

If *V. vulnificus* enters through a wound, the skin around the wound can break down, causing the same skin lesions as with ingestion.

Whether by ingestion or wound contamination, *V. vulnificus* infection without rapid and aggressive treatment can result in a mortality rate of 50% in people with preexisting conditions such as liver disease (e.g., hepatitis C), hemochromatosis, kidney disease related to transplants, diabetes mellitus, cancer (lymphoma, leukemia, and Hodgkin's disease), stomach disorders, or a

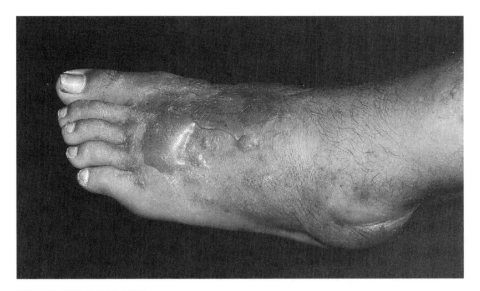

FIGURE 50. Blistering lesions caused by *Vibrio vulnificus*. (Courtesy C Samlaska, MD. From James WD, Berger TG, Elston DM: *Andrews' diseases of the skin clinical dermatology*, ed 10, Philadelphia, 2006, Saunders.)

suppressed immune system. In immunocompetent people there are usually no lasting complications once the disease has resolved itself.

DIAGNOSIS

Diagnosis starts with a history of eating shellfish, mollusks, fin fish, or a wound exposed to seawater and the clinical signs and history. *Vibrio spp.* can be cultured from feces, blood, or fluid from skin lesions.

TREATMENT

Uncomplicated *V. parahaemolyticus* infection in immunocompetent people usually does not require medical intervention as the vibriosis resolves. Maintaining fluids in people with diarrhea is important. Antibiotics do not seem to lessen the severity of the diarrhea or shorten the recovery period.

V. vulnificus septicemia infections need to be treated with antibiotics immediately to increase the chances of patient survival. The wounds must be aggressively debrided. Amputation may be necessary to stop the spread of the infection. Even with aggressive treatment, the mortality rate can reach 50% in people with preexisting conditions.

PREVENTION

There is no vaccine for vibriosis prevention. There is no way to eliminate the *V. parahaemolyticus* and *V. vulnificus* organisms because they are part of the normal marine environment. Cooking shellfish thoroughly and avoiding saltwater areas when wounds are present are two of the best ways to prevent vibriosis. Other important precautions follow:

- Do not eat oysters or other shellfish raw.
- Boil shellfish until the shells open, and then 5 minutes more.
- Steam shellfish until the shells open, and then 9 minutes more.
- Do not eat shellfish that do not open during cooking.
- Boil shucked oysters for at least 3 minutes.
- Fry shucked oysters in oil at least 10 minutes.
- Fry fish until the thickest part is opaque.
- Do not eat raw fish. Even though most cases of vibriosis result from ingesting contaminated shellfish, precautions should be taken when eating raw fish, especially with the current popularity of sushi and sashimi.
- Do not cross-contaminate other food with raw shellfish juices or raw seafood.
- Wear gloves when handling raw shellfish or seafood.
- Do not expose open wounds, broken skin, or burns to warm seawater.
- Keep raw shellfish and seafood away from open wounds and broken skin.

WEST NILE VIRUS INFECTION

West Nile virus (WNV) infection is more widespread throughout North America than any of the other equine encephalitides. WNV was originally identified in Europe, Africa (Uganda), the Middle East, and western Asia. In 1999 the first case of WNV infection was reported in the United States. How it got to North America is unknown.

MORBIDITY:+
MORTALITY: ++
ETIOLOGY: VIRAL

WNV is the arbovirus (*arthropod-borne virus*) that causes WNV infections. Other arboviruses include the eastern equine encephalitis virus, western equine encephalitis virus, La Crosse encephalitis virus, and St. Louis encephalitis virus.

HOSTS

Hosts include vertebrates: over 100 species of birds, horses, and humans.

TRANSMISSION

Migratory birds play an important role in the spread of the virus. Common sparrows are resistant to the effects of WNV and are therefore considered natural reservoirs for the virus. Crows and blue jays are severely affected by the virus, and the presence of dead crows or blue jays may indicate the presence of WNV in an area. WNV is spread by the bite of an infected mosquito (Figure 51). Horses and humans are infected when a mosquito takes a meal from an infected bird and subsequently bites a horse or human. Horses, humans, and other mammals do not develop a level of virus in the blood that is significant enough to make them a source of infection to other animals via a mosquito bite; they are, therefore, considered dead-end hosts.

WNV infection is indirectly zoonotic, meaning humans and horses cannot be infected directly from one another or from birds. The mosquitoes act as vectors that transmit the virus. WNV infection occurs most commonly from late spring through early fall, when mosquitoes are most active.

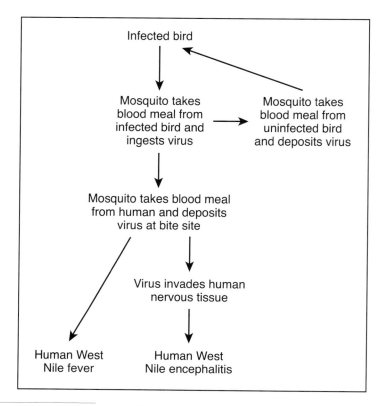

FIGURE 51.   West Nile virus infection.

In humans there have been rare cases of transmission of WNV through organ transplants, blood transfusions, breast feeding, and through the placenta during pregnancy.

WEST NILE VIRUS INFECTION IN HORSES

Most infected horses will not become clinically ill. If an infected horse becomes clinically ill, the signs are related to the inflammation in the brain, or *encephalitis*, caused by the virus. These include nonspecific signs such as loss of appetite, depression, and fever. The encephalitis can be manifested by difficulty swallowing, weakness or paralysis of a hind limb, impaired vision, incoordination, head pressing, aimless wandering, walking in circles, excitability, convulsions, coma, and death. These signs will usually appear between 5 and 15 days after infection. Animals usually recover in 4 to 7 days and do not show any signs of permanent brain damage. The mortality rate in horses can be up to 33%.

Not all animals showing clinical signs of encephalitis are infected with WNV. Other diseases associated with encephalitis include rabies, botulism, and eastern and western equine encephalitis.

WEST NILE VIRUS INFECTION IN HUMANS

WNV infection in humans will usually be asymptomatic or will only cause mild symptoms. About 20% of the people infected will develop a mild illness known as *West Nile fever*. West Nile fever is characterized by fever, headache, fatigue, muscle aches, and sometimes a rash on the chest, stomach, and back. The incubation period is from 5 to 15 days, and the illness lasts 3 to 6 days.

In less than 0.02% of people infected with WNV, a severe and sometimes fatal neuroinvasive infection will develop. It can involve only the membranes covering the brain (meninges), or it can involve the entire brain (encephalitis). Meningitis is characterized by headaches, high fever, and neck stiffness. Encephalitis causes a more severe disease characterized by fever, headache, disorientation, muscle tremors, blindness, numbness, paralysis, convulsions, coma, and death. The encephalitis is more severe in people over 50. Symptoms can last several weeks, and if the person recovers, there may be permanent brain damage. Over half the people who die from the encephalitis are more than 77 years old.

DIAGNOSIS

Initially diagnosis is based on clinical signs and time of year. A final diagnosis is made by virus isolation, from the brain tissue of dead humans or animals, and serologic testing.

TREATMENT

There is no specific antiviral drug treatment for WNV infection. Supportive therapy, such as administration of nutritive fluids, medications to decrease brain swelling, and antibiotics to treat or prevent secondary bacterial infections, may make the patient more comfortable.

PREVENTION IN HORSES

Prevention of WNV infection in horses involves vaccination and decreased exposure to mosquitoes. There is no evidence that WNV infection can be transmitted directly between horses, between humans, or between horses and humans.

Reducing exposure to mosquitoes involves the following precautions:

- Drain areas of standing water. These are mosquito breeding sites.
- Keep horses inside during peak mosquito activity, from early evening until after dawn.
- Keep lights off in stables during the night. Mosquitoes are attracted to incandescent lights.
- Put screens on stable windows and keep fans blowing to prevent mosquito access.
- Place incandescent lights around the outside of the stable to attract mosquitoes and keep them away from horses.
- Fog the stable with an approved pesticide in the evening.
- Use mosquito repellents intended specifically for horses.

A number of vaccines are available that protect against WNV infection; these should be administered by a veterinarian, following the manufacturer's guidelines. Horses that have been vaccinated against eastern and western equine encephalitis are not protected against WNV infection.

PREVENTION IN HUMANS

Prevention of WNV infection in humans involves decreased exposure to mosquitoes. There is no vaccination available for protection against WNV infection in humans.

Reducing exposure to mosquitoes involves the following precautions:

- Drain areas of standing water, especially after rainfall and watering. These are mosquito breeding sites.
- Reduce outdoor activities during peak mosquito activity.
- Wear protective clothing when mosquitoes are most active, especially in the early evening and early morning. Protective clothing includes long-sleeved shirts and long pants.
- Use insect repellent containing DEET on exposed skin.
- Make sure screens fit properly and do not have any holes to decrease mosquito access to building interiors.

WESTERN EQUINE ENCEPHALITIS

Western equine encephalitis is a viral disease of horses and humans. It is seen mostly west of the Mississippi River in the United States and in corresponding provinces in Canada.

MORBIDITY: +
MORTALITY: +
ETIOLOGY: VIRAL

Western equine encephalitis virus (WEEV) is an arbovirus (*arthropod-borne virus*) that causes Western equine encephalitis. Other important encephalitis arboviruses include the eastern equine encephalitis virus, St. Louis encephalitis virus, La Crosse encephalitis virus, and West Nile virus.

HOSTS

Hosts include vertebrates, especially birds, humans, and horses. The natural hosts for WEEV are passerine birds, such as blackbirds, finches, jays, sparrows, and warblers.

TRANSMISSION

WEEV is found mainly in or near farmland or irrigated fields and is transmitted through the bite of an infected mosquito (Figure 52). Horses and humans are infected when a mosquito takes a meal from an infected bird and subsequently bites a horse or human. The mosquito deposits the virus in the blood when it feeds. Horses and humans do not develop a level of virus in the blood significant enough to make them a source of infection to other animals via a mosquito bite; they are, therefore, considered dead-end hosts.

WEE is *indirectly zoonotic*, meaning humans and horses cannot be infected directly from one another or from birds. The mosquito acts as a vector, transmitting the virus. WEE occurs most commonly from late spring through early fall, when mosquitoes are most active.

WESTERN EQUINE ENCEPHALITIS IN HORSES

WEE is a central nervous system disease in horses, but the disease is not as severe as the one caused by EEEV. The clinical signs of WEE, seen from 5 days

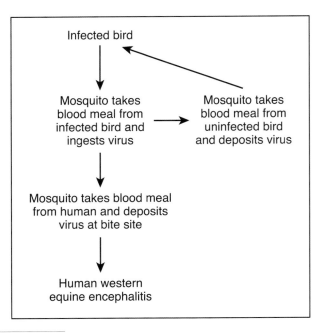

FIGURE 52.   Western equine encephalitis.

to 3 weeks after infection, include fever, depression, anorexia, sensitivity to light, staggering, circling, disorientation, paralysis, and death. Even though WEEV is considered less pathogenic than EEEV, the mortality rate for animals showing clinical signs can reach 20% to 50%. Animals that are not severely affected by WEE recover in a couple of weeks, but permanent brain damage, especially abnormal reflexes, may remain.

WESTERN EQUINE ENCEPHALITIS IN HUMANS

Human WEE cases are usually first seen in June or July. In most WEE cases, the infections are either asymptomatic or cause a mild, nonspecific disease. Clinical signs include fever, headache, stiff neck, nausea, vomiting, anorexia, and fatigue, followed by central nervous sytem signs that may include paralysis, abnormal reflexes, coma, and death. Children under 1 year old and young adults are more severely affected than other age groups. Recovery may be accompanied by permanent brain damage in 5% to 30% of young patients. Most adults recover in 7 to 10 days without permanent brain damage. The mortality rate in infected humans is 3% to 15%.

DIAGNOSIS

Initially diagnosis is based on clinical signs, season, and geographic location. A final diagnosis is made by virus isolation from the brain tissue of dead horses or humans or serology testing for the presence of antibodies against WEEV.

TREATMENT

There is no specific antiviral drug treatment for WEE. Supportive therapy, such as administration of nutritive fluids, medications to decrease brain swelling, and antibiotics to treat or prevent secondary bacterial infections, may make the patient more comfortable.

PREVENTION IN HORSES

Prevention of WEE in horses involves vaccination and decreased exposure to mosquitoes. There is no evidence that the WEEV can be transmitted between horses, between humans, or between horses and humans.

Reducing exposure to mosquitoes involves the following precautions:
- Drain areas of standing water. These are mosquito breeding sites.
- Keep horses inside during peak mosquito activity, from early evening until after dawn.
- Keep lights off in stables at night; mosquitoes are attracted to incandescent lights.
- Put screens on stable windows, and keep fans blowing to prevent mosquito access.
- Place incandescent lights around the outside of the stable to attract mosquitoes and keep them away from horses.
- Fog stables with an approved pesticide in the evening.
- Use mosquito repellents intended specifically for horses.

Vaccines are available for protection against WEEV infection and should be administered in the spring. Initial vaccination requires multiple injections, which are followed by annual boosters.

PREVENTION IN HUMANS

Prevention of WEE in humans involves decreased exposure to mosquitoes. There is no vaccination available to prevent WEE in humans.

Reducing exposure to mosquitoes involves the following precautions:
- Drain areas of standing water. These are mosquito breeding sites.

- Reduce outdoor activities during peak mosquito activity.
- Wear protective clothing when mosquitoes are most active, especially in the early evening and early morning. Protective clothing includes long-sleeve shirts and long pants.
- Use insect repellent containing DEET on exposed skin.
- Make sure screens fit properly and do not have any holes. This will decrease mosquito access to building interiors.

YERSINIOSIS

Yersiniosis is a bacterial disease that usually affects the intestinal tract. The disease is seen most often in young children and during the cooler months of the year, usually November through January.

MORBIDITY: +
MORTALITY: +
ETIOLOGY: BACTERIAL

Yersiniosis is caused by a gram-negative rod, *Yersinia enterocolitica*. Some readers may recognize the genus name from *Yersinia pestis*, the causative agent of the plague. These two bacteria belong to the same genus but cause different diseases.

Y. enterocolitica needs iron to survive, so the more iron a person has in the blood, the more *Y. enterocolitica* may grow. This becomes important in diseases that are characterized by elevated iron levels, such as hemochromatosis, sickle cell disease, and thalassemia.

Y. enterocolitica grows best in an environment that is slightly alkaline. People taking antacids that reduce stomach acidity are creating more alkaline environments in their intestinal tracts, which creates more favorable growing conditions for *Y. enterocolitica*.

Cool temperatures favor the growth of *Y. enterocolitica*, which is why yersiniosis is seen more often during the cooler, winter months.

HOSTS

Y. enterocolitica is found in the feces of many animals. Pigs are the most common source of human infection. Other strains that can cause human disease are found in dogs, cats, rodents, rabbits, horses, cattle, and sheep. Once infected, a person will shed the *Y. enterocolitica* organism.

TRANSMISSION

Most people will get infected by eating feces-contaminated food or by drinking contaminated milk or water. Undercooked or raw pork is a common source of infection. Preparing chitterlings, made from the small intestines of pigs, can be especially dangerous.

Unpasteurized milk and dairy products and untreated water can also be contaminated with *Y. enterocolitica*. The organism has also been found in cold cuts, ice cream, tofu, and shellfish from contaminated water, lakes, and streams.

Infants can be infected if caregivers are not meticulous about washing their hands after handling raw meat or after using the bathroom. The organism can be passed from the caregiver to anything infants put in their mouths, which could be just about anything within reach.

Other sources of *Y. enterocolitica* can include produce contaminated with raw manure containing *Y. enterocolitica*, direct contact with infected animals, and cross-contamination of food preparation utensils and cutting surfaces.

YERSINIOSIS IN ANIMALS

Most animals that shed *Y. enterocolitica* appear clinically healthy. Some animals will have mild diarrhea or frequent stools covered with mucus or blood. Many cases of yersiniosis may go undiagnosed because veterinarians are not looking for the disease and because laboratories do not routinely culture for *Y. enterocolitica* unless it's specifically requested.

YERSINIOSIS IN HUMANS

Yersiniosis in people can range from an asymptomatic disease to overwhelming septicemia and death. Adult patients seem to develop a less severe disease.

Young children will usually develop a fever, accompanied by abdominal pain and diarrhea with or without mucus or blood. The incubation period is 4 to 7 days. Most children will recover without treatment in 1 to 3 weeks. In severe cases, the bacteria may pass through the intestinal wall and enter the blood stream, producing septicemia. These cases usually require hospitalization and antibiotic treatment.

Older children and young adults frequently develop the same symptoms. The abdominal pain is more acute in the lower right abdominal quadrant and is often confused with appendicitis.

In rare cases in older patients, complications can arise when infections are found outside the intestines. There may or may not be septicemia associated with these infections. The most common complications are skin rash, which is more common in women, and joint pain, especially in the knees. These conditions can appear up to a month after the initial infection and usually clear up without treatment.

DIAGNOSIS

Yersiniosis is diagnosed by culturing a stool sample for the presence of *Y. ente-rocolitica*. Laboratories must be asked specifically to culture for the *Y. enterocolitica* organism, which has also been found in the throat, lymph nodes, joint fluid, urine, bile, and blood.

Serologic testing can detect the presence of antibodies against *Y. enterocolitica*.

TREATMENT

Treatment is usually not necessary unless severe septicemia develops. The most important aspect of recovery is to keep patients hydrated while they have diarrhea. *Y. enterocolitica* is susceptible to many antibiotics. Some patients have mistakenly had their appendix removed based on the acute, abdominal pain on the right side.

PREVENTION

Yersiniosis can be prevented by following these precautions:
- Thoroughly cook all meat, especially pork, before eating it.
- Observe all "keep refrigerated," "sell by," and "use by" warnings on food labels.
- Wash hands, cutting surfaces, and utensils that come in contact with raw meat.
- Drink only pasteurized milk or products made from pasteurized milk.
- Avoid feces-contaminated water.
- Wash all produce before eating it.
- Meticulously wash hands after handling raw meat, especially pork. *This is very important when making chitterlings*. Hands and fingernails need to be scrubbed thoroughly after handling pig intestines. It would probably be wise to have someone not involved in chitterling preparation care for infants.
- Wash hands after using the bathroom or changing diapers.
- Wash hands after handling animals. This is very important if the animal has diarrhea.
- Properly dispose of animal feces.

Life Cycle of a Tick

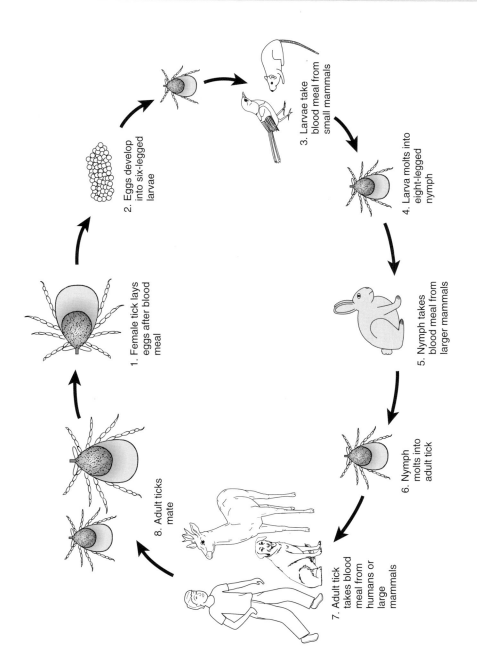

1. Female tick lays eggs after blood meal

2. Eggs develop into six-legged larvae

3. Larvae take blood meal from small mammals

4. Larva molts into eight-legged nymph

5. Nymph takes blood meal from larger mammals

6. Nymph molts into adult tick

7. Adult tick takes blood meal from humans or large mammals

8. Adult ticks mate

appendix two

Identification of Ticks

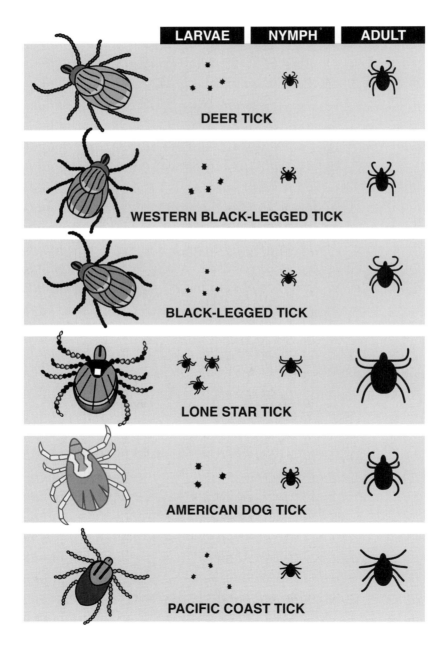

	LARVAE	NYMPH	ADULT
DEER TICK			
WESTERN BLACK-LEGGED TICK			
BLACK-LEGGED TICK			
LONE STAR TICK			
AMERICAN DOG TICK			
PACIFIC COAST TICK			

appendix three

How to Protect Yourself Against Ticks

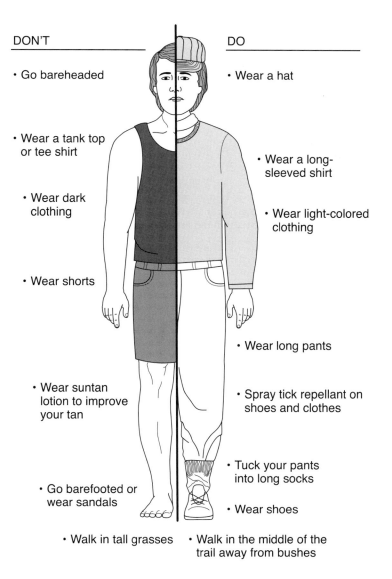

DON'T | DO

DON'T
- Go bareheaded
- Wear a tank top or tee shirt
- Wear dark clothing
- Wear shorts
- Wear suntan lotion to improve your tan
- Go barefooted or wear sandals
- Walk in tall grasses

DO
- Wear a hat
- Wear a long-sleeved shirt
- Wear light-colored clothing
- Wear long pants
- Spray tick repellant on shoes and clothes
- Tuck your pants into long socks
- Wear shoes
- Walk in the middle of the trail away from bushes

Tick Removal Procedure

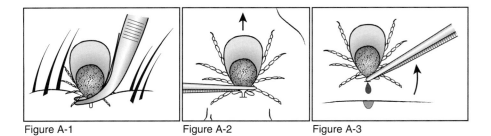

Figure A-1   Figure A-2   Figure A-3

1. Grasp the tick with pointed tweezers as close to the skin as possible (Figure A-1).

2. Using slow, steady, firm force, pull the tick in the reverse direction in which it is inserted (Figure A-2).

3. Maintain pressure until the tick can be pulled from the skin. This may take some time. Do not pull back quickly or with jerky movements (Figure A-3). This could result in the body being separated from the head, which will remain embedded in the skin. If this happens, remove the head like you would a splinter.

4. Don't squeeze the tick while it's still attached. This could force more infective fluid into the wound.

5. Do NOT apply petroleum jelly, fingernail polish, fingernail polish remover, repellents, pesticides, or a lighted match to an attached tick. They may irritate the tick to force more liquid into the wound, and they are ineffective tick removal methods.

6. Place the tick in a small, clean container that contains alcohol. Seal the container. Alternatively, place the tick in a small, clean container that can be sealed (e.g., jar or baggie) and put it in the freezer. This will preserve the tick if it has to be identified later.

7. Wash the wound and your hands with warm soapy water. Apply antiseptic to the wound.

NOTE: The preserved ticks can be discarded after 1 month. All known tick-borne diseases will display symptoms within a month.

• It can take hours to days before pathogens are transmitted from the tick to the host, so ticks should be removed as soon as possible.

• For optimum safety, latex gloves should be worn for tick removal.

appendix five

The 4 Cs of Food Safety

1. Clean
   - Clean hands—always wash your hands with warm soapy water before handling food.
   - Clean utensils and preparation surfaces—wash all utensils, cutting boards, or other surfaces with warm soapy water if they come in contact with raw food. This means any raw food, not just meat.
   - Clean raw vegetables and fruits before eating them.

2. Cook
   - Cook meat thoroughly. Ideally there should be no pink in the middle.
   - Cook leftovers until they are hot throughout.

3. Cover
   - Cover food when it is not being served or eaten.
   - Partially cover leftover food and put it in the refrigerator to cool.
   - Cover leftovers when they cool.

4. Chill or Heat
   - Food poisoning bacteria grow best between 41° F (5° C) and 140° F (60° C). Perishable food needs to be kept outside this danger zone to prevent food poisoning.

212° F/100° C
High temperatures destroy most bacteria

165° F/73° C
Low cooking and holding temperatures prevent growth but allow some bacteria to live

140° F/60° C
DANGER ZONE:
Rapid growth of bacteria; some will produce toxins

40° F/4.44° C

32° F/0° C
Water freezes

0° F/−18° C
Freezer setting

glossary

abscess - accumulation of pus accompanied by inflammation

alopecia - loss of hair

anorexia - loss of appetite

arbovirus - arthropod-borne virus

bradyzoite - slowly growing stage in the growth of some parasites

cachexia - weight loss and wasting of muscle

cellulitis - inflammation of the subcutaneous or connective tissue

chorioretinitis - inflammation of the choroid membrane and retina

congenital - present at birth

conjunctivitis - inflammation of the conjunctiva (mucous membrane of eyelid and eyeball)

dyspnea - difficulty breathing

edema - accumulation of fluid in tissues

encephalitis - inflammation of the brain

endocarditis - inflammation of the lining of the heart

enteritis - inflammation of the intestinal tract, especially the small intestine

eosinophilia - increased number of eosinophils in blood

erythema - redness of the skin, often a sign of inflammation or infection

eschar - dry scab on the skin

gastroenteritis - inflammation of the mucous membranes of the stomach and intestines

hemoglobinuria - hemoglobin in the urine

hepatomegaly - enlarged liver

hydrocephalus - accumulation of fluid in the ventricles of the brain

jaundice - yellowish discoloration of eyes, skin, and mucous membranes; icterus

laminitis - inflammation of tissue in the hoof of a horse

lethargy - sluggishness, apathy

lymphadenopathy - enlargement of lymph nodes

malaise - vague feeling of discomfort, unease

mastitis - inflammation of the udder

meningitis - inflammation of the membranes covering the brain and spinal chord

microcephaly - smaller than normal head

myalgia - muscular pain or tenderness

necropsy - autopsy of a dead animal

necrosis - death of tissue

necrotizing fasciitis - death of skin and muscle due to bacterial toxins

ophthalmia - inflammation of the eye, especially the conjunctiva

osteomyelitis - inflammation of bone and bone marrow, usually due to infection

PCR - polymerase chain reaction; a means of detecting specific kinds of DNA or RNA

paresthesia - tingling, burning, or itching skin sensation with no apparent cause

pericarditis - inflammation of the membrane covering the heart

polyuria - excessive production and passing of urine

purulent - having, discharging, or causing the production of pus

pustule - small swelling of skin, such as a pimple or blister

septicemia - invasion of the bloodstream by pathogenic organisms or their toxins

splenomegaly - enlarged spleen

tachypnea - rapid breathing

tachyzoite - rapidly multiplying, asexual stage of some parasites

viremia - presence of virus in the blood

Index